W9-BWZ-836

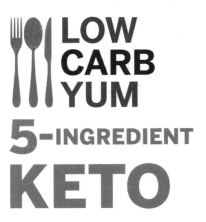

LOW
CARB
YUM

5-INGREDIENT

KETO

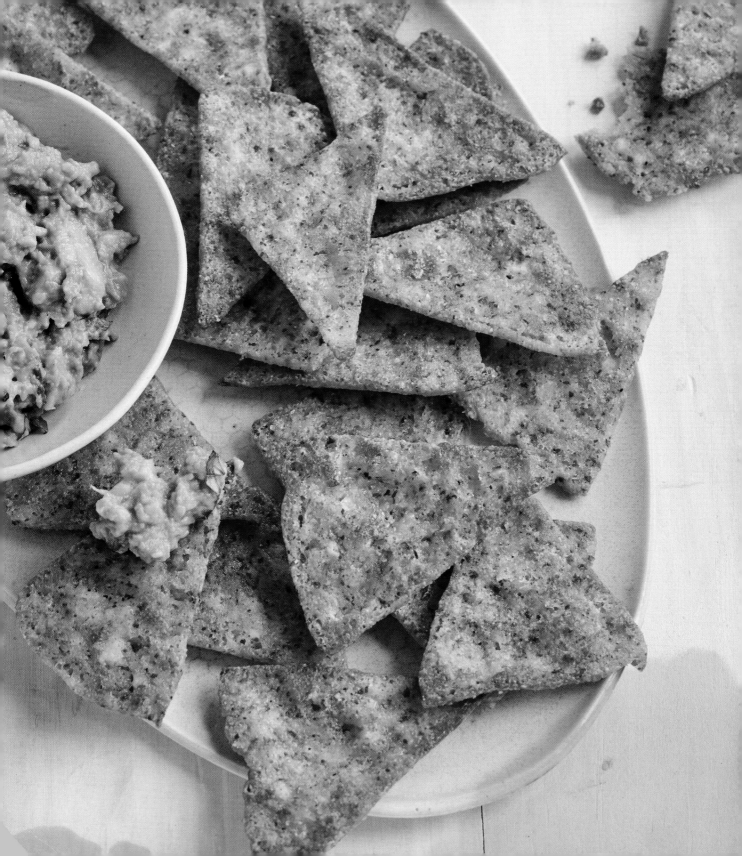

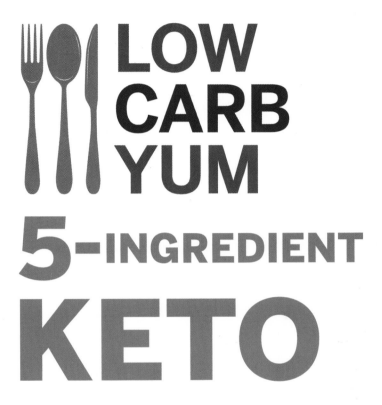

LOW CARB YUM

5-INGREDIENT KETO

LISA MARCAURELE

Founder of Low Carb Yum

PHOTOGRAPHY BY LAUREN VOLO

HOUGHTON MIFFLIN HARCOURT
BOSTON NEW YORK 2020

Copyright © 2020 by Lisa MarcAurele

Photography copyright © 2020 by Lauren Volo

Food styling by Monica Pierini

Prop styling by Maeve Sheridan

Kitchen illustrations: Zarian/Depositphotos and Lub Lubachka/Depositphotos

For information about permission to reproduce selections from this book, write to trade .permissions@hmhco.com or to Permissions, Houghton Mifflin Harcourt Publishing Company, 3 Park Avenue, 19th Floor, New York, New York 10016.

hmhbooks.com

Library of Congress Cataloging-in-Publication Data

Names: MarcAurele, Lisa, author. | Volo, Lauren, photographer.
Title: Low carb yum 5-ingredient keto : 120+ easy recipes / Lisa MarcAurele, founder of Low Carb Yum ; photography by Lauren Volo
Description: Boston : Houghton Mifflin Harcourt, 2020. | Includes index. | Summary: "Incredibly easy recipes from Low Carb Yum, one of the all-time most popular low-carb and keto blogs"— Provided by publisher.
Identifiers: LCCN 2019040536 (print) | LCCN 2019040537 (ebook) | ISBN 9780358237020 (trade paperback) | ISBN 9780358229230 (ebook)
Subjects: LCSH: Ketogenic diet. | Reducing diets. | Low-carbohydrate diet. | LCGFT: Cookbooks.
Classification: LCC RM237.73 .M36 2020 (print) | LCC RM237.73 (ebook) | DDC 641.5/6383--dc23
LC record available at https://lccn.loc.gov/2019040536
LC ebook record available at https://lccn.loc.gov/2019040537

Book design by Jan Derevjanik

Printed in China

SCP 10 9 8 7 6 5 4 3 2 1

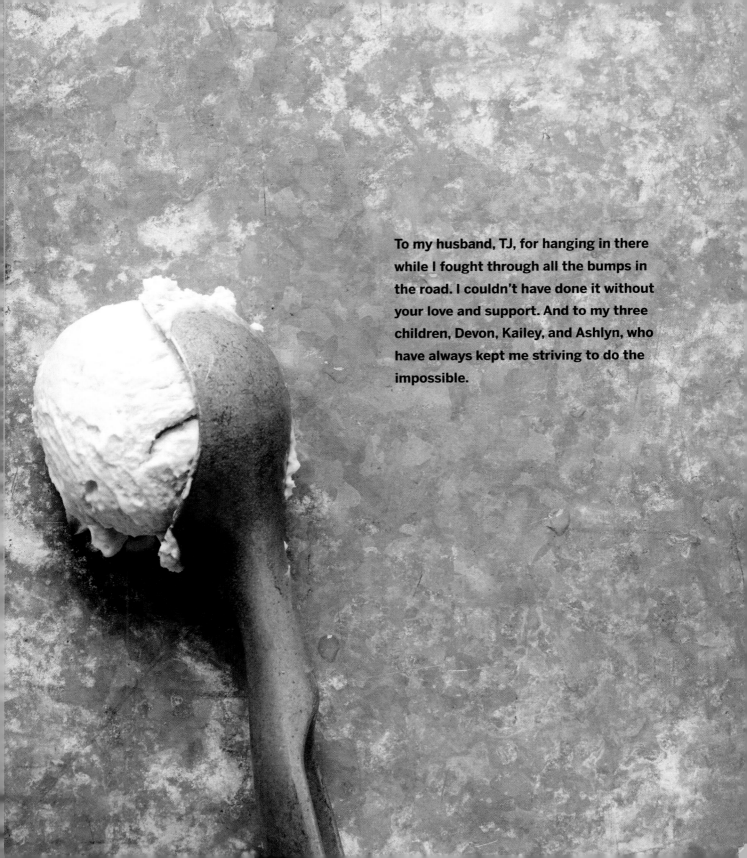

To my husband, TJ, for hanging in there while I fought through all the bumps in the road. I couldn't have done it without your love and support. And to my three children, Devon, Kailey, and Ashlyn, who have always kept me striving to do the impossible.

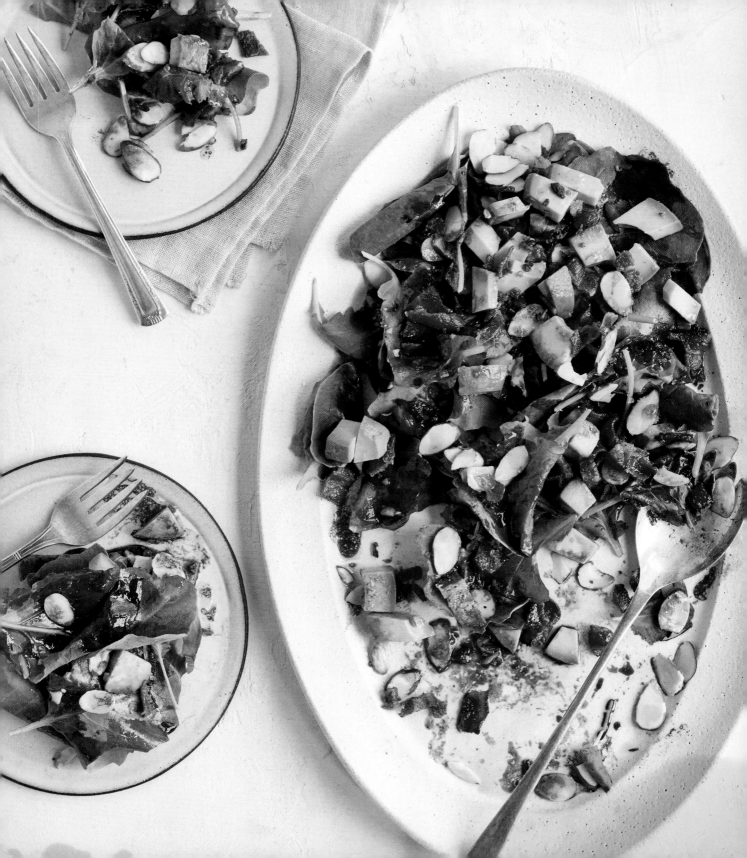

CONTENTS

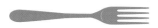

ACKNOWLEDGMENTS ix

INTRODUCTION

MY STORY xii
BASICS ON A LOW-CARB AND KETO DIET xiv
HOW TO GET STARTED xviii
SAMPLE DAILY MEAL PLANS xxxi

BREAKFAST

Almond Flour Pancakes 2
Scrambled Eggs with Crabmeat 4
Cauliflower "Mock" Porridge 5
Spinach-Tomato-Avocado Omelet 7
Granola Cereal 8
Bacon-Egg Cups 10
Minute Muffin 11
Coconut–Almond Butter Bars 13
Bagel Thins 14
Coconut Flour Waffles 17
Egg Casserole with Sausage and Spinach 18
Breakfast Burrito 20
Broccoli-Cheddar Egg Muffins 21
Breakfast Pizza 23

SOUPS AND STEWS

Slow-Cooked Roasted Bone Broth 26
Broccoli-Cheese Soup 27
Sausage-Kale Soup 28
Chicken Zoodle Soup 31
Egg Drop Soup 32
Oyster Stew 34
No-Bean Chili 35
Creamy Avocado Soup 37
Cabbage and Ground Beef Soup 38
Cream of Mushroom Soup 40
Pumpkin Soup 41
Yellow Squash Soup 43
Roasted Brussels with Bacon Soup 44
Chicken Chili 47

SALADS

Baby Vegetable Mixed Salad 50
Creamy Dill-Cucumber Salad 52
Broccoli Salad 53
Summer Squash Salad 53
Radish Salad 56
Sour Cream–Lettuce Salad 57
Baby Kale Salad 58
Wedge Salad 58
Spinach-Bacon Salad 61
Green Bean–Tomato Salad 62
Salmon-Cucumber Salad 64
Cabbage Salad 65
Pesto Chicken Salad 67

APPETIZERS AND SNACKS

Almond Flour Bread 70
Almond Cheese 72
Mexican Cheese Dip 73
Nutty Crackers 76
Stuffed Cucumber Slices 77
Cheese Ball 78
Avocado Deviled Eggs 79
Seasoned Tortilla Chips 80
Sour Cream and Onion Dip 83

DRESSINGS AND SAUCES

Italian Dressing 86
Avocado Dressing 86
Chocolate Sauce 87
Strawberry Sauce 87
Maple Syrup 88
Avocado Mayonnaise 89
Cheese Sauce 92
Basil Pesto 92
Balsamic Vinaigrette 93
Blue Cheese Dressing 94
Low-Carb Ketchup 95

SIDE DISHES

Fried Spinach with Mushrooms 98
Stir-Fried Squash and Pepper 101
Fried Cabbage with Bacon 102
Wilted Lettuce with Bacon 104
Cauliflower Mash 105
Turnip Fries 106
Mushrooms Provençale 107
Sautéed Celery 107
Pork Fried Rice 109
Roasted Broccoli 110
Almond Asparagus 111
Creamed Spinach 114
Sautéed Red Cabbage 114
Walnut Zucchini 115

MAIN DISHES: POULTRY AND PORK

Roasted Chicken 118
Garlic-Lemon Chicken 120
Chicken-Broccoli Casserole 121
Broccoli and Cheese Stuffed Chicken 123
Baked Chicken Thighs 124
Curried Chicken 127
Marinated Turkey Tenderloins 128
Smothered Pork Chops 129
Filipino Chicken Adobo 130
Ham and Collard Greens 133
Egg Roll in a Bowl 134
Pork Loin Roast 136
Chicken with Spinach and Tomato 137
Quick "Breaded" Pork 139

MAIN DISHES: BEEF AND LAMB

Rib-Eye Steaks in Red Wine Sauce 142
Beef Filet with Mushrooms 144
Zucchini Meatloaf 145
Lamb Patties 147
Ginger Beef and Asparagus 148
Ground Beef and Cabbage 150
Pepper Steak 151
Beef Pot Roast 153
No-Noodle Lasagna 154
Stuffed Peppers 156
Cheeseburger Casserole 157
Steak Pinwheels 159

Garlic Lamb Chops 160
Braised Short Ribs 163

MAIN DISHES: SEAFOOD

Fish Florentine 166
Salmon with Creamy Dill Sauce 166
Crab Quiche 169
Shrimp Scampi 170
Stir-Fried Scallops 173
Garlicky Steamed Mussels 174
Baked Flounder with Tomato 177
Balsamic Halibut 178
Tuna Casserole 179
Butter Fish 180
Creamy Clam Sauce over Zoodles 181
"Breaded" Flounder 182

DESSERTS

Crustless Baked Cheesecake 186
Fluffy Strawberry Cream 189
Vanilla Custard Pudding 190
Raspberry-Cheese Muffins 191
Coconut Macarons 192
Chocolate Fudge Balls 195
Quick Ricotta Pudding 195
No-Churn Vanilla Ice Cream 196
Baked Coffee Custard 198
Coconut Milk Pudding 199
Almond Butter Cookies 201
Chocolate Mousse 202
Almond Flour Cake 205
Almond Butter Cups 206

BEVERAGES

Keto Coffee or Tea 210
Almond Milk 210
Green Tea Smoothie 211
Raspberry Smoothie 211
Golden Milk 215
Hot Cocoa 215
Strawberry Milkshake 216
Strawberry Lemonade 216
Ginger-Turmeric Tea 218

INDEX 219

ACKNOWLEDGMENTS

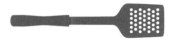

A special thanks to my editor, Justin Schwartz, whose knowledge and experience made this cookbook possible. It's been a pleasure working with you and the amazing team that you assembled. I really enjoyed working with the photography team that created all the incredible recipe photos. Thank you, Lauren Volo, Monica Pierini, and Maeve Sheridan.

I'd also like to thank my agent, Stacey Glick, for all her help getting this project off the ground.

Thank you to my husband, TJ, for taking care of everything at home so I could devote time to this book project along with the tasks needed to maintain the Low Carb Yum website. I couldn't have done any of this without you.

Special thanks to my three children: My daughter Kailey for helping me keep up with tedious blog tasks. My son, Devon, for giving my recipes a try and letting me know how they tasted. And my daughter Ashlyn for keeping me company in the kitchen.

I'd like to thank my father for showing me how to cook basic dishes when I moved into my first college apartment over 1,000 miles away from home. And a thank-you to my mother for giving me my very first cookbook, which taught me various cooking techniques and will always be the favorite in my collection. A big thanks to my sister Nesa for spreading the word about Low Carb Yum with all her coworkers. And I appreciate all the support from my sister Donna, and brothers Ray and John. My sister Mary also deserves a special mention even though she lost her battle with cancer before I started blogging. Her illness is one of the reasons I decided to move to a low-carb eating plan for good.

A thank-you to my husband's parents and sister, who have inspired many of my recipes through family gatherings that have always included a wide variety of foods.

I'm especially thankful for the work that my assistant, Pie, has done over the years. Without her, I wouldn't have been able to keep up with everything. I'd also like to thank Chantal, Holly, Jovita, Marci, Lisa Yvonne, Bec, Thena, and Piper for taking care of tasks that I didn't have time to do myself.

A big thanks to all those in the blogging community who have helped me grow my blogging hobby into a thriving business. I've met so many wonderful people it would be impossible to name them all.

And last, but certainly not least, I'd like to thank all those who have supported the Low Carb Yum blog over the years, with a special mention to Vickie, who has become a top fan.

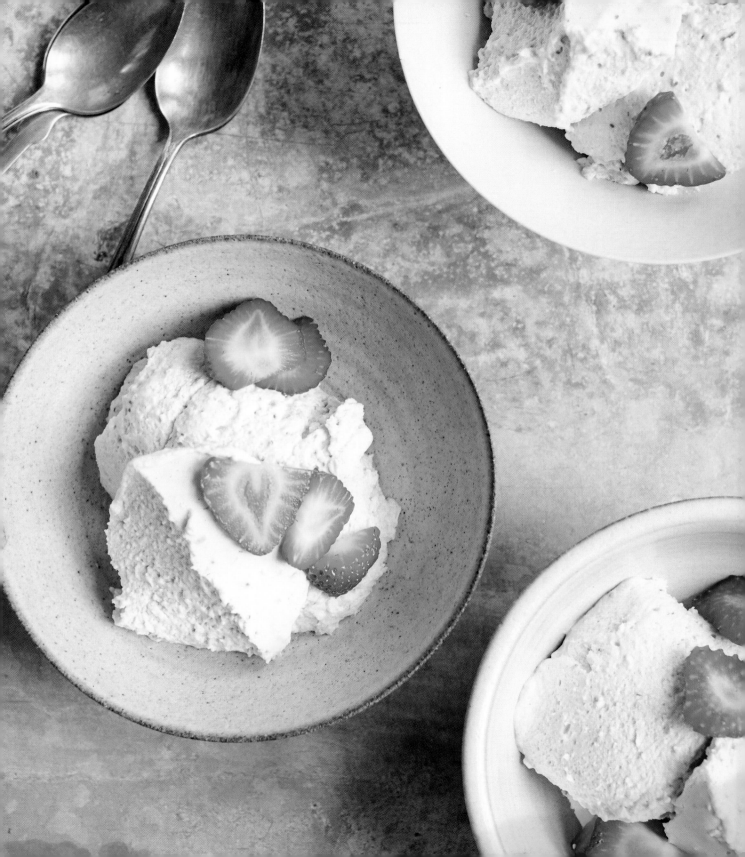

INTRODUCTION

MY STORY

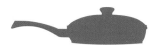

IMAGINE BEING ABLE TO EAT WHATEVER YOU want and not gain any weight. High-carb? Low-carb? No-carb? Doesn't matter. This was my reality. My metabolism used to be in constant overdrive, allowing me eat anything I wanted and not put on an ounce of fat. Jealous?

Don't be. You see, the guilt-free buffet didn't last very long. In my mid-twenties, my thyroid was treated with radioactive iodine. With no more overactive thyroid keeping my metabolism high, I started gaining weight quickly.

Now, before I tell you how I was able to lose the unwanted weight, let me explain why I decided on this treatment. After all, you're probably wondering why I would purposely mess with my metabolism.

Blame it on the autoimmune condition called Graves' disease. I was diagnosed with Graves' shortly after the birth of my first child. Unlike many people who struggle with an underperforming thyroid, Graves' is the exact opposite problem. Although I had a revved-up metabolism, there are plenty of unpleasant symptoms that come along with the disease, like bulging eyes and severe anxiety. After a few years of unsuccessful interventions, including antithyroid medication that didn't control my condition, I reluctantly gave my doctor permission to destroy my thyroid.

After my thyroid was irradiated, my eating habits were the same as before the treatment: high-carb and high-calorie. No wonder I was putting on so much weight rapidly. Desperate to stop the weight gain, I began to try different weight loss approaches. The standard method of counting calories and cutting fat didn't work for me. All it did was leave me hungry and miserable because the food wasn't satisfying.

I had heard about people losing incredible amounts of weight by eating high-fat foods like bacon, eggs, and cheese. The only catch was that carbohydrates had to be significantly cut back. Being an engineer, I wanted to know the science behind a low-carb diet, so I began reading as many books as I could about the subject.

Back then, I wasn't much of a cook, so I bought some books with low-carb recipes. But there weren't many cookbooks specializing in low-carb, so I began to experiment in the kitchen, adapting some of my favorite recipes into low-carb versions. I began to learn how to substitute low-carb ingredients for the high-carb staples that I had relied on. However, because I worked long hours and had a busy family life, I fell off the low-carb wagon and reached the heaviest weight of my life. Thankfully, with a change in jobs came a more normal, stress-free schedule. Shortly after the job change, I made a commitment to lose the excess weight.

Low-carb, here I come (again). But this time, it won't be just a temporary diet; it will be a lifelong lifestyle, I promised myself. Enter SugarFreeLowCarbRecipes.com, a website I started in 2010. My intention in creating it was using it both as an online food journal to help me stay on track and as digital storage for the recipes I was creating. I ended up losing all the extra weight within the first year of blogging! The site name eventually changed to LowCarbYum.com in January 2015, but the content remained the same.

I could never have imagined that over the course of the next decade, my blog would help millions of people from all over the world be successful with a long-term low-carb eating plan. I am humbled that the feedback I've received shows that not only is it helping people stick to a low-carb plan, people are thriving and loving these low-carb recipes.

My motto is "keep it simple," so I tend to favor quick-and-easy recipes that don't take much effort to prepare. To make things even easier, this cookbook provides over 130 simple recipes that use just 5 ingredients or less. Why? Because minimal ingredients make grocery shopping easier and simplify preparation. (It should be noted that oil for frying and salt and pepper are not counted in the ingredient count since they are standard cooking items. I also didn't count optional ingredients.)

Following a low-carb eating plan has been the key to maintaining a healthy weight for me while enjoying satisfying real-food meals. My recipes are all gluten-free, grain-free, keto-friendly, and made without any added sugar. And many of the recipes can be made with dairy-free alternatives, so you'll find tons of paleo-friendly recipes as well.

Low-carb eating has completely changed my life. I hope that my *Low Carb Yum 5-Ingredient Keto* cookbook will help make a positive change in your life too!

LISA

BASICS ON A LOW-CARB AND KETO DIET

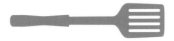

What Is Low-Carb?

For the most part, a low-carb diet is any eating plan that restricts carbohydrates to 100 grams or less of total carbohydrates per day. Some plans even go as high as 150 total carbs a day, but for those who are looking for maximum weight loss, eating less than 50 grams per day is the most effective limit because it causes the body to go into a state of ketosis.

What Is Ketosis?

Ketosis is when the body uses fat instead of glucose for energy. Carbohydrates are converted into glucose, so significantly cutting back on eating carbohydrates should force the body into a state of ketosis. While in ketosis, fat is broken down to make glucose in the liver, and fatty acids known as ketones are created as a by-product of the process.

To determine the degree of ketosis, your body's ketone levels can be measured. The most accurate method is to test blood levels using a meter that can measure both glucose and ketones. There are also urine strips and breathalyzers available; however, urine tests basically test excess ketones that pass as waste and many breathalyzers are inaccurate. Be sure to check out the reviews before buying any product to determine if it will provide an accurate measurement of ketosis.

What Is a Low-Carb Diet?

There are three general categories of low-carb diets, which are grouped by the daily total carbs consumed:

LIBERAL (100–150 GRAMS CARBS): Active people with a high metabolic rate can usually lose weight by cutting carbs to less than 150 grams per day. This is also a range that can be used for maintaining weight, especially for more active people.

MODERATE (50–100 GRAMS CARBS): People who don't have a lot of weight to lose or prefer a slow and gradual approach find success with a moderate low-carb eating plan. Staying in the range of 50–100 grams per day is also a great way to maintain weight long term.

STRICT (<50 GRAMS CARBS): Those looking to lose weight quickly will need to be very strict and keep carbs to less than 50 grams a day. This is also the range needed to maintain ketosis.

When I first started on the low-carb lifestyle, I followed a strict plan with less than 50 grams a day. But after reaching my weight loss goal, I gradually moved to a moderate plan. Since my thyroid condition puts my metabolism on the slower end and I don't do a lot of intense exercise, staying under 100 grams a day is a good range for maintaining my weight. However, when I find the scale starting to creep up, I move myself to a stricter keto diet.

What Is a Keto Diet?

The keto diet has become the most popular low-carb plan, but it may not be the best diet for everyone. That's because it's the most strict, and some may find it difficult to adhere to the optimal daily amounts of carbs, protein, and fat.

The goal of the keto diet is to maintain a state of ketosis. For many people, ketosis can be achieved by reducing carbohydrates to anything less than 50 grams a day. However, some people find they need to decrease carb limits to as low as 20 to 30 grams a day and maintain a deeper state of ketosis in order to lose weight.

Daily Macros

When following a keto diet, there are optimal daily macronutrient (*macro* for short) percentages that one should target. These typically fall into the following ranges:

Fat: 65–80 percent

Protein: 15–30 percent

Carbs: 5–10 percent

Personally, I find the most difficult part of the keto diet is continuously monitoring the macro percentages for each day. To make this easier, there are a number of keto diet apps that can be installed on a smartphone or tablet, but you'll need to track everything you're eating, which takes some discipline.

Another thing to keep in mind is that many recipes only state the amount of carbohydrates, protein, and fat in grams and not percentages. Fortunately, if you know how to do the math, it's easy to calculate percentages yourself. You can make it even easier by putting the formulas into a spreadsheet like Microsoft Excel or Google Sheets.

Here are the formulas to do the calculations yourself:

NET CARBS = Total Carbs − Fiber Carbs − Non-impacting Sugar Alcohol Carbs

% CARBS = Net Carbs × 4 / Calories

% PROTEIN = Protein × 4 / Calories

% FAT = Fat × 9 / Calories

CALORIES = (Net Carbs × 4) + (Protein × 4) + (Fat × 9)

Note that when calculating the percentage of carbohydrates, the fiber carbs aren't counted in the standard calculation. Net carbs are used instead of total carbs because fiber isn't easily digested. Therefore, fiber carbs shouldn't impact blood sugar in the same way as other carbohydrates. Since it's poorly digested and not readily available for the body to use as energy, calories from fiber are ignored.

Some argue that the digestion of fiber depends on whether it's soluble or insoluble. Soluble fibers are either absorbed or dissolved by water and are able to be digested by bacteria. Because of this slower digestion, they typically provide about half the calories as regular carbohydrates, or roughly 2 calories per gram. Insoluble fibers, however, aren't digested at all, so they don't provide any calories. Therefore, insoluble fiber can be completely removed by the equation, whereas half the soluble fiber should be counted.

How do you know if the fiber you are eating is soluble or insoluble? It's not easy, as most plants contain both types of fiber. Foods high in soluble fiber are black beans, Brussels sprouts, avocados, broccoli, and flaxseeds. Whereas wheat bran, whole grains, berries, spinach, radishes, as well as the skin of most fruits and vegetables tend to be high in insoluble fiber. If you're unsure whether the fiber is soluble or insoluble, it's best to count half the fiber carbs in the net. To be on the safe side, you may want to count net carbs using the following:

NET CARBS = Total Carbs – ½ Fiber Carbs

However, since subtracting all the fiber carbs is standard practice for calculating net carbs, the macro percentages for the recipes in this book do not include fiber. If you'd rather include the fiber, I recommend using an app that allows you to choose tracking either net carbs or total carbs. That way you can track the total carbs that you are consuming each day based on the foods you are eating.

When following a keto diet, fat should account for just under 75 percent of your total calories, while protein makes up about 20 percent. The remaining 5–10 percent of your calories will come from carbohydrates. A lot of people struggle with eating enough fat to meet the target daily percentage because health authorities have told us to avoid fat for so long. With the majority of calories coming from fat on keto, you'll need to eat plenty in order to not go over on carbs and protein. However, you don't want to overdo the fat either, as it's calorie-dense. You do need to watch your calories too, which is something I'll discuss in the next section.

Here are a couple of suggestions to get in some fat without adding additional carbs or protein:

- If the food you're eating is low in fat, be sure to add in a healthy fat. For example, you'll want to top off steamed vegetables with butter and use a high-fat dressing in a tossed salad.

- You can drink a hot coffee or tea with a tablespoon of coconut oil or butter blended in. This great for satisfying hunger when you've reached your daily limit on both carbs and protein, but still have haven't reached the calories and fat allotted for the day.

It's easy to consume too much protein when cutting back on carbs. But if adequate fat is consumed, there's no need to fill up on protein. That's because fat is very filling and curbs the appetite. Many find that when following a ketogenic diet, they can go much longer between meals. Some even practice intermittent fasting, in which the time between finishing dinner and starting breakfast is extended. This practice lengthens the overnight fast to around 16 hours and allows for a deeper state of daily ketosis.

What About Calories?

Although you're not required to count calories, it's good to have an idea of how many calories you should be consuming each day. This number is based on your gender, weight, height, age, and activity level. To determine daily calories needed to maintain your current weight, you just take your basal metabolic rate (BMR), or calories needed daily while resting, and multiply it by your activity factor.

BMR IS CALCULATED AS FOLLOWS USING THE MIFFLIN-ST. JEOR BMR EQUATIONS:

MALES:
$(4.536 \times$ body weight in lbs$) + (15.88 \times$ height in inches$) - (5 \times$ age$) + 5$

FEMALES:
$(4.536 \times$ bodyweight in pounds$) + (15.88 \times$ height in inches$) - (5 \times$ age$) - 161$

THE ACTIVITY FACTORS ARE:

SEDENTARY
(little or no exercise): 1.2

LIGHTLY ACTIVE
(light exercise/sports 1–3 days/week): 1.375

MODERATELY ACTIVE
(moderate exercise/sports 3–5 days/week): 1.55

VERY ACTIVE
(hard exercise/sports 6–7 days a week): 1.725

EXTRA ACTIVE
(very hard exercise/sports at least twice daily or a physical job): 1.9

EXAMPLE

Here's how a 35-year-old woman who's 63 inches tall, weighs 145 pounds, and is lightly active would calculate her daily calorie target:

BMR $= (4.536 \times 145) + (15.88 \times 63) - (5 \times 35) - 161 = 1322.16$

DAILY CALORIES FOR MAINTENANCE = BMR $\times$ Activity Factor $= 1322.16 \times 1.375 = 1{,}818$ calories

If you want to lose weight, you should be consuming fewer calories than what's needed to maintain your weight and/or upping your activity to burn more calories. With a low-carb ketogenic diet, people tend to eat fewer calories than needed. This is because the calories consumed are primarily from fat, which is very filling, so it's easier to eat fewer calories each day. However, I find that keeping daily calories at least 500 calories below daily maintenance is best for weight loss. Also note that as you lose weight, the calories for maintenance will go down, so your daily calorie consumption will need to go down as well as you become lighter.

The calculations involved with following a keto diet properly can make your head spin if you constantly have to do them manually. That's why I always use a keto diet app on my cell phone to track my daily macros easily and accurately when I want to lose weight.

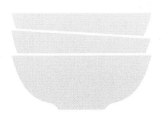

HOW TO GET STARTED

YOU'VE DECIDED TO TRY LOW-CARB OR KETO.
Now what? The first thing is to make sure you have the right mind-set. It's got to be something you really want to do, and you need to have a clear image of what you want to achieve. Whether it's losing weight or improving health, you must set an attainable and measurable goal to focus on. You also need to commit to the plan and be willing to change your lifestyle for good.

For those new to low-carb, it's best to start out by using a food journal so you can track everything you're eating. When I returned to low-carb in 2010, I used a popular weight loss app to keep track of everything I ate. The program made sure I had the calorie deficit needed to meet my weight loss goals, but that app wasn't specific to low-carb, so it didn't track my optimal daily targets for carbs, protein, and fat. However, with keto being so popular these days, there are a ton of keto diet apps that have a lot more features and are specially designed for getting the right daily macro percentages.

After a week or two of keeping a food journal, you'll begin to learn when you should eat, how much of each food to eat, and what you shouldn't eat. You'll also learn how to consume the ideal macronutrient (fat, protein, carbs) ratio for each meal. If journaling becomes too tedious, you can try a few days without it and see how it goes. For the best results, though, I recommend continuing to keep track of what you're eating until you reach your goal. It's easy to go off track if you aren't using some kind of food journal to keep yourself accountable for the things you're eating.

Foods to Eat

Those new to the keto diet will need to take some time to become familiar with what foods are allowed and which ones aren't. Unfortunately, many people still believe that fat is bad for you, but healthy fats from whole foods should *not* be avoided on a ketogenic diet. These fats not only provide more flavor, but they are also satisfying and will keep you full longer. Following a keto diet will naturally make you eat less because it helps to suppress hunger better between meals.

When shopping for food, you may notice that whole foods tend to be found on the perimeter of the grocery store. Since processed foods often come in bags, boxes, and cans, they are usually placed in the aisles. I find that shopping for low-carb foods is easier because only a few items that I need are located in the middle of the store. Things such as canned meat, cooking oil, vinegar, canned low-carb vegetables, coffee, tea, and seasonings are found in the aisles.

Learning what foods to eat is the most important part of transitioning to low-carb eating. That's why I've provided a handy list to make it easier.

MEAT · Pretty much all beef, chicken, pork, lamb, and game meats are acceptable. With poultry, it's best to go for skin-on leg pieces, which have less protein and more fat.

SEAFOOD · When choosing fish, go for fatty fish high in omega-3s that still have the skin on. Crab, mussels, scallops, shrimp, lobster, squid, and octopus are also good options.

EGGS • Any type of egg is appropriate. Large chicken eggs are standard for recipes, but duck and quail eggs can be eaten too. I've experimented with duck eggs and found they make low-carb baked goods turn out fluffier.

VEGETABLES • There are many choices when it comes to vegetables, but generally, it's best to choose those that grow above ground. Leafy greens like spinach and lettuce have the least amount of carbs. Other popular choices are asparagus, eggplant, zucchini, cucumber, cabbage, kale, cauliflower, and broccoli.

NUTS • The best nuts are pecan, macadamia, and Brazil nuts because they have the fewest net carbs. Hazelnuts, walnuts, almonds, and pine nuts can also be consumed. Some people avoid peanuts because they are technically a legume that's eaten like a nut, but peanuts can be enjoyed in moderation. Coconut is often grouped with nuts, but it's not a true nut and is considered more of a fruit. Coconut is also a keto-friendly food.

SEEDS • Chia, flax, sunflower, sesame, and pumpkin seeds fit well into a ketogenic diet plan.

FATS • The best fats to use are olive oil, coconut oil, avocado oil, butter, ghee, and lard. Avoid vegetable and seed oils, which are unstable fats prone to oxidation, meaning they then turn rancid easily.

FRUITS • Savory fruits like avocados, olives, and tomatoes are best since they have the least amount of sugar. For sweet fruits, stick to berries like unsweetened cranberries, strawberries, blackberries, raspberries, and blueberries. Coconut can also be enjoyed as a sweet fruit.

DAIRY • Full-fat cheese and cream are allowed on a low-carb diet. Some Greek-style yogurts are ultra-filtered to remove milk sugar and can be keto-friendly. However, regular milk shouldn't be consumed because a one-cup serving has about 12 grams of total carbs. It should also be noted that sometimes dairy can hinder weight loss. Therefore, those with a lot of weight to lose may want to try going dairy-free. Those with an autoimmune disease may want to avoiding dairy as well, because milk proteins can aggravate the inflammatory condition.

PASTA ALTERNATIVES • The easiest way to replace noodles is to use a spiralizer device to prepare vegetables like zucchini, yellow summer squash, or spaghetti squash. (Many markets also sell these vegetables pre-cut in this way.) If using them in a dish like lasagna, it's best to remove as much of the liquid as possible so the dish doesn't turn out watery. Spiralized zucchini is my favorite noodle substitute, but shirataki noodles made from konjac root fiber are also a popular keto option.

THICKENERS • When it comes to making things like homemade gravy, you may want to add a keto-friendly ingredient to thicken the sauce. Xanthan gum and guar gum are popular in low-carb recipes, but I prefer not to use them because they can aggravate autoimmune conditions. Instead I prefer using glucomannan, which is a water-soluble fiber that comes from the root of the konjac plant. It's the same fiber used to make shirataki noodles.

FLOURS · You'll want to keep almond flour and coconut flour in your pantry. Other flours you may want to consider (especially if you have an allergy to almond or coconut) are peanut flour, flax meal, and sesame seed flour. Psyllium husks are also great for making low-carb breads. If you can't find some of these nut or seed flours, it's easy to finely grind nuts or seeds into a flour using a coffee grinder or small blender.

SWEETENERS · Erythritol, stevia, and monkfruit are the most popular natural sweeteners. Other natural sweeteners that can be used include xylitol, allulose, kabocha extract, and prebiotic fibers like inulin. Artificial sweeteners like sucralose, saccharin, acesulfame potassium, and aspartame can also be used, but they are more controversial and may have negative side effects.

A Few Things to Note about Keto Foods . . .

The digestible carbohydrates in vegetables, nuts, seeds, and fruits need to be carefully monitored if you're following a keto diet with less than 20 grams of net carbs a day. It's easy to overeat vegetables when on a very strict low-carb diet. Stick to vegetables that have less than 5 grams of net carbs per serving. Nuts and seeds are easy to overeat, so be sure to consume them in moderation. Fruits should also be limited or avoided on keto.

Sweeteners, which will be discussed in more detail later, should not be overly relied upon. Occasional treats are fine, but they shouldn't replace wholesome foods like meats, eggs, and vegetables. Although there are sweeteners that have zero carbs or zero net carbs, consuming them in excess can have a negative impact on appetite control and body weight.

Foods to Avoid

Learning what foods to avoid is just as important as knowing what foods to eat. Below you'll find a list of items to remove from your diet:

- Things with white or wheat flour
- High-sugar fruits and fruit juice
- Anything with added sugars
- Rice and other grains
- Starches like potatoes
- Most legumes like beans (peanuts and soy may be okay)
- Higher-carb nuts like cashews and pistachios
- Packaged foods with net carb claims that are also high fiber (the fiber is often soluble)
- Sugar alcohols other than erythritol and xylitol
- Sweeteners with high-carb fillers like maltodextrin

To resist tempting foods, I recommend purging your kitchen of all the foods you need to avoid.

Common Mistakes

The keto diet is very effective for losing weight. However, sometimes it may not be working as well as expected. In this section, you'll find ten common mistakes that can cause weight loss stalls and sometimes even lead to weight gain.

1 NOT RESTRICTING CARBS ENOUGH

For the best chance of ketosis, carbohydrates should be limited to less than 50 grams per day. If not using an accurate measurement system, it's easy to go overboard with carbs. Another problem is eating a portion that's larger than a serving. It can help to measure or weigh food in the beginning to make sure the portion sizes are accurate

If counting net carbs, restricting yourself to 20 grams net carbs or less a day is usually effective. Keep in mind that what works for others may not work for you. And it's always best to count total carbs, especially with packaged foods where you may be unsure if the fiber is soluble or insoluble.

If you are new to keto and don't have a feel for what it takes to get into and maintain a state of ketosis, start by using a mobile app on your cell phone to track everything you're eating. There are many programs available so pick one that works best for you. This will allow you to easily track progress and use the data to determine the daily macros that work best for your body.

2 GOING BY THE SCALE

After transitioning to a carb-restricted diet, the majority of the weight loss in the beginning is from water. That's why many people tend to see a huge amount of weight shed at the start, but then the weight loss slows down and may stall.

Taking measurements of your waist, hips, and chest and recording them in a journal can be a good way to track progress. You can take measurements each week, every other week, or once a month. Weight should also be taken at similar intervals. You may notice that your body measurements are going down even if the scale isn't moving. Some keto apps have the option to track body measurement as well as daily macros so you can monitor your progress.

If exercise or strength training has been started at the same time, muscle mass may be building as fat goes down. Keep that in mind if you are sticking to the plan but not seeing your weight go down.

3 TOO MUCH DAIRY

Overindulging in low-carb dairy products can cause weight loss stalls. That's because whey protein has been shown to stimulate the pancreas to produce insulin. Increased insulin levels will make getting into ketosis difficult. If you suspect this may be happening, avoid dairy products that contain whey, like heavy cream and yogurt. Butter doesn't contain much protein so it's usually okay, and hard cheeses have most of the whey removed.

The casein in milk products can also be a problem. The protein in cheese is mainly casein so it may need to be avoided. But there's two types of casein: A1 and A2. Most cow milk has a mix of both. However, the A1 form has been shown to trigger gut inflammation and digestive issues, so consuming dairy containing only A2 casein is typically best, as excess inflammation can hinder weight loss. It's often difficult to find low-carb A2-only dairy products, but there are some online companies that sell them if you can't find them locally. The casein in sheep and goat milk is the A2 kind, so products made with those types of milks are always an option too.

 4 NOT STAYING HYDRATED

Drinking a lot of water during the day is needed to flush out excess ketones and burn fat more efficiently. It's also believed that water helps break down fat more efficiently. Also, consuming adequate water is one way to stay full without consuming food and calories. I find that drinking at least 16 ounces of water instead of eating is a great way to curb hunger.

Another benefit of drinking a lot of water on a keto diet is that it helps relieve constipation and flu-like symptoms when first transitioning to a low-carbohydrate eating plan. The recommended amount is at least 8 cups, or 64 ounces, of water every day.

LACK OF EXERCISE

Exercising isn't required to lose weight on a keto diet, but it will help you shed the weight more efficiently. That's because restricting carbohydrates encourages releasing fat from storage to be used as energy. However, if there's no activity to burn this source of energy, the fat may just go back into storage.

Too much exercise can cause unnecessary stress to the body, so it's not a good idea to jump into a high-intensity workout right away. This is especially true if you haven't been very active before moving to keto. It's best to take a gradual approach and work your way into the more strenuous routines. A leisurely bike ride or taking brisk walks after lunch or dinner are perfect ways to get moving!

 TOO MANY PACKAGED FOODS

When starting out on keto, don't run out and buy all those keto products you see online and in local stores. Stay away from the ones that contain ingredients you wouldn't use in your own kitchen. They may help with weight loss, but the net carb claims can be misleading. Many add fiber sweeteners that aren't from soluble fiber sources to make the products taste good. In other words, some of those carbs subtracted from the net carb count may still be having an impact!

It's best to get your daily carb allowance from whole foods like fresh vegetables, fruits, and nuts. These foods are much more nutritious than any keto bar or shake that comes in a package.

EATING TOO MANY SWEETS

Although berries are low in carbs, the sugar in them can cause weight-loss stalls or even lead to weight gain. Stick to only a small handful of berries at a time and consume them in moderation.

The same goes for low-carb sweeteners. Even though they are sugar-free and calorie-free it's best not to consume too much because they may negatively affect your appetite. Artificially sweetened foods have been shown to trigger hunger, which can lead to overeating.

 CONSUMING A LOT OF CALORIES

It's true that a keto diet isn't a calorie-restricted diet. However, that doesn't mean you should be consuming more calories than needed. Overeating on any diet is likely to cause weight gain. It's a good idea to track calories and keep them well under the daily amount needed to maintain your current weight. This is especially important if the weight isn't coming off as expected. Consuming adequate fat and drinking plenty of water should keep hunger under control while restricting calories and carbs.

 GOING OVERBOARD WITH FAT

Even though keto is a high-fat diet, it's important to only eat the amount of fat needed. If the fat consumed isn't used as energy, it could get stored instead. This is particularly true if you are consuming too many calories from fat. It's a good idea to use one of the various keto calculators available online to determine how much fat you should be eating each day. Keto apps also have a keto calculator built in to help you determine the optimal amount of protein, fat, carbs, and calories you should be consuming each day.

 NOT MONITORING BLOOD SUGAR

If the thought of pricking your finger to take a blood sample makes you uneasy, you may want to skip this. However, I've found that glucose meters are a great way to determine if certain foods impact ketosis. (There are even blood meters available that measure ketone levels to help determine your state of ketosis!) Glucose meters are available in local pharmacies. They are the best way to accurately determine if certain foods cause your blood sugar to rise. And when your blood sugar rises, your body releases insulin, which can trigger fat storage and knock you out of ketosis.

OTHER THINGS TO CONSIDER

If you've gone through this list and none of the items apply, it may be time to check with your doctor. Hormonal imbalances and other conditions may be getting in the way of weight loss. Thyroid disorders are a common cause of slow weight loss. If your thyroid has tested to be within the normal range and you still think there may be a problem, ask your doctor to test your thyroid antibody levels. Testing antibodies can pick up on autoimmune thyroid disease like Hashimoto's disease much earlier than standard thyroid testing.

All About Sweeteners

Breaking a sugar addiction can be difficult, but there are a lot of keto-friendly sweeteners to help make the transition to a sugar-free diet easier. However, I recommend avoiding sweeteners as much as you can. I find that they can slow weight loss and lead to overeating. People who resist sweets while on an eating plan to lose weight typically have more success than those who regularly eat sweetened foods.

A study at the University of Sydney ("Why artificial sweeteners can increase appetite," 13 July 2016, https://sydney.edu.au/news-opinion /news/2016/07/13/why-artificial-sweeteners-can -increase-appetite.html) discovered that consuming the artificial sweetener sucralose led to consuming more calories than needed. The study concluded that when sweetness versus energy (calories) is out of balance, the brain responds with a stimulated appetite to consume more calories. Keep in mind that even though these low-carb sweeteners may have zero calories, the sweet taste can trigger cravings for more sweets or more food in general.

When I indulge in foods sweetened with zero-calorie sweeteners, even natural sweeteners, I tend to overeat and consume more calories than I need. Because sweets seem to trigger hunger for me, I get the best weight loss results if I avoid sweets altogether. It's much better to fill up on moderate-protein high-fat meals than to eat a sweetened keto meal replacement bar.

NATURAL SWEETENERS

When I do use sweeteners, I prefer natural ones. However, even though these sweeteners are derived from plants, they must undergo processing to create a usable sweetener. Other than dried ground stevia leaves, all low-carb sweeteners are man-made through some kind of processing. Some refer to all processed sweeteners as "fake sugars" regardless of whether they are natural or artificial.

When I first started on low-carb, I had to rely on artificial sweeteners, as natural ones weren't easy to find. But these days, there are a lot of choices. I've listed the natural based keto sweeteners that I've tried below.

ERYTHRITOL · A sugar alcohol is usually made from fermented corn sugar, erythritol is often used in ketogenic recipes because it's been shown to have no effect on blood sugar or insulin level. Therefore, carbs free from erythritol are not included in net carbs. And unlike other sugar alcohols, it typically doesn't cause digestive issues like gas and bloating if eaten in moderation. One downside is that it has a "cooling effect" because of its cool minty aftertaste, but blending erythritol with other sweeteners like stevia and/or monkfruit can lessen that. It's only 70 percent as sweet as sugar, so blending it with a stronger sweetener creates a one-for-one sugar replacement.

STEVIA · This herbal sweetener is extracted from the leaves of the *Stevia rebaudiana* plant. To make stevia sweetener, processing is done to isolate the glycosides, which are the sweet compounds found in the leaves. To extract the glycosides, the stevia leaves must go through an extensive chemical process. Unprocessed, dried ground stevia leaves are available, but they have a grassy taste that many people don't care for. I find the dried leaves are perfect for tea and other beverages. Stevia can also have a bitter aftertaste, but some processing methods are able to remove this undesirable taste to make it more palatable.

MONKFRUIT · Sometimes referred to as *lo han guo*, monkfruit is a gourd-like fruit that's similar in size to a lemon. But it's a fruit that's rarely eaten fresh because it's hard to store and has undesirable flavors. The Chinese use the fruit dried, but often combine it with a sweetener to offset the bitter flavor. Chemical processing is able to isolate the sweet part of the fruit. The sweetener extract is very similar to stevia, but tends to have a more pleasant taste.

ALLULOSE · Gaining popularity in the keto community is a rare sugar called allulose that measures zero on the glycemic index and is about 70 percent as sweet as regular sugar. It can be made from corn or fruit sugar using a special enzyme conversion process. The nice thing about allulose is that although it doesn't raise blood sugar, it has properties very similar to standard white sugar. It's not calorie-free, though. One gram of the sweetener contains about one-third of a calorie. Because of its sugarlike qualities, it can give keto ice cream and low-carb cookies the texture they are often missing when other sweeteners are used.

PREBIOTIC FIBERS · Prebiotics are carbohydrates, but they don't get digested. Instead, they pass into the colon where they feed beneficial bacteria. Since they are slightly sweet, they can be used as low-carb sweeteners. There are two main types of prebiotics: inulin and oligofructose. They are found in many vegetables and other plants. Inulin is usually produced from chicory root and oligofructose is a component of inulin that can be isolated using an enzymatic process. Potential benefits of fiber sweeteners are improved gut health and lowered appetite. Inulin is often combined with other sweeteners because it's only about 35 percent as sweet as sugar. A downside of inulin is that it can have a laxative effect and cause cramping if too much is consumed. It's also not a good choice for baking since it can degrade above 275°F.

XYLITOL · This sugar alcohol is found in fruits and vegetables. It's as sweet as sugar but with only 40 percent of the calories. However, it often causes gas and bloating. It also needs to be kept away from animals like cats and dogs, as it can be lethal to them in small doses. The net carbs tend to be high (60g per 100g), and consuming it may impact ketone production. Therefore, it's best to avoid it on a keto diet.

TAGATOSE · This simple sugar occurs naturally in dairy, fruits, and cacao. The lactose from whey in cow's milk is typically used to isolate the sweetener. It has a slightly cool aftertaste similar to erythritol. It's 75 to 90 percent as sweet as sugar, but with less than 40 percent of the calories. With a low glycemic index of 3, it only has a small impact on blood glucose and insulin levels. Some brown sugar replacements use it because it caramelizes like sugar. It needs to be used in moderation, though, as it contains more carbs than other options (about 35g net carbs per 100g).

KABOCHA EXTRACT · A relatively new sweetener that extracts pentose from kabocha, a winter squash often referred to as Japanese pumpkin. Kabocha extract has zero calories and measures zero on the glycemic index. The carbs are from pentose, which is metabolized for energy without the use of insulin. It does have a sweet taste similar to sugar without any aftertaste and has been shown not to impact blood sugar. However, there isn't a lot of research on the use of kabocha extract as a sweetener so use it in moderation until more information is available.

MIRACLE FRUIT (MIRACULIN) · You may not have heard of miracle fruit, but it's a berry native to West Africa that makes sour and acidic foods taste sweet. It contains a compound known as miraculin, which is a taste modifier that binds to the taste buds stimulating the sweet receptor cells. The effect is temporary and usually lasts for about 30 minutes, but some claim it can last more than an hour. The berries can be purchased frozen, freeze-dried, powdered, or in tablets. Although it can be added to foods, it's popular to dissolve miracle fruit on the tongue before eating. With miracle fruit, you may be able to leave out the sweetener and just dissolve a tablet in your mouth before enjoying an unsweetened dessert!

MY EXPERIENCE WITH NATURAL SWEETENERS

I find that combining natural sweeteners provides the best overall taste. Many of my recipes on LowCarbYum.com use a combination of sweeteners rather than just one. My favorite blend is stevia and monkfruit extracts, but I've found that with some recipes, especially when baking, erythritol or another bulk sweetener is often needed too. My preference is to use an erythritol–monkfruit blend with stevia extract mixed in. This not only provides the best overall taste, but also cuts back on the amount of erythritol used. Adding monkfruit extract to an erythritol stevia blend does the same thing.

ARTIFICIAL SWEETENERS

With so many natural low-carb sweeteners, there's no need to use synthetic ones, and some studies indicate that certain artificial sweeteners can have negative effects like stimulating the appetite. I recommend sticking to natural sweeteners but will go over some of the synthetic sweeteners and mention why I avoid them.

SUCRALOSE · The popular artificial sweetener in the yellow packets is sucralose. It's created by chlorinating sugar to replace three hydroxyl groups with three chlorine atoms. Recent studies show that sucralose breaks down when heated, so it isn't a good choice for baking as it can release potentially toxic chemicals. It's also been shown to increase appetite, which can result in overeating. However, if you do choose to use sucralose, I recommend sticking to the liquid version, which doesn't contain any high-carb fillers. Also be sure to use it only for non-cooked items.

SACCHARIN · The sweetener in the pink sugar substitute packets is usually saccharin. It's not commonly used these days because animal-based testing concluded it was potentially a cancer-causing substance. Saccharin can also have an undesirable bitter taste, especially when cooked.

CYCLAMATE · Because it's only 30 to 50 times as sweet as sugar, cyclamate is often combined with saccharin. Mixing the two sweeteners has a synergistic effect making the blend taste much better by toning down the undesirable flavors found in each. A benefit of cyclamate is that it's stable when heated. However, safety concerns have led to it being banned in the United States and other countries. It remains approved for use in Canada, the European Union, and other places.

ACESULFAME POTASSIUM (K) · One benefit that acesulfame K has over other artificial sweeteners is that it's stable under heat. It has a bitter aftertaste, though, which is why it's often blended with another sweetener. It has been shown to negatively affect the gut bacteria and body weight in animal studies (https://www.ncbi.nlm.nih.gov/pmc/articles/PMC5464538/), so it's best to avoid.

ASPARTAME · Commonly found in the blue sweetener packets and in diet soft drinks, aspartame is a widely used artificial sweetener. However, it isn't recommended for baking as it can break down and become bitter with an undesirable aftertaste. There's also a lot of reports linking the artificial sweetener to cancer, headaches, weight gain, and other potential ailments.

SWEETENER CONVERSION CHART FOR NATURAL KETO SWEETENERS

Sugar	1 tsp	1 Tbsp	¼ cup	⅓ cup	½ cup	1 cup
Erythritol	1¼ tsp	1 Tbsp + 1 tsp	⅓ cup	⅓ cup + 2 Tbsp	⅔ cup	1⅓ cups
Stevia (powder)	⅟₃₂ tsp	⅟₁₆ + ⅟₃₂ tsp	⅜ tsp	½ tsp	¾ tsp	1½ tsp
Stevia (liquid)	5 drops	15 drops	½ tsp	⅔ tsp	1 tsp	2 tsp
Monkfruit (powder)	⅟₆₄ tsp	⅟₃₂ + ⅟₆₄ tsp	⅛ + ⅟₁₆ tsp	¼ tsp	¼ + ⅛ tsp	¾ tsp
Monkfruit (liquid)	8 drops	24 drops	¾ tsp	1 tsp	1½ tsp	3 tsp
Allulose	1¼ tsp	1 Tbsp + 1 tsp	⅓ cup	⅓ cup + 2 Tbsp	⅔ cup	1⅓ cup
Inulin	1 Tbsp	3 Tbsp	¾ cup	1 cup	1½ cups	3 cups
Xylitol	1 tsp	1 Tbsp	¼ cup	⅓ cup	½ cup	1 cup
Tagatose	1 tsp	1 Tbsp	¼ cup	⅓ cup	½ cup	1 cup
Kabocha extract	1 tsp	1 Tbsp	¼ cup	⅓ cup	½ cup	1 cup

Note: Conversion can vary by brand, especially for stevia and monkfruit extracts. For example, some liquid monk fruit is 4 drops to replace a teaspoon of sugar, so all measurements for those brands would be half of what is shown. A "pinch" measuring spoon can be used for ⅟₁₆ tsp and a "smidgen" measure can be used for ⅟₃₂ tsp.

Removing Inflammatory Foods

After years of struggling to maintain my weight with a dysfunctional thyroid, I've discovered that carbohydrates are only part of the problem. When it comes to health issues like diabetes, autoimmune disease, and obesity, there's more to the story than just cutting back on processed foods and carbohydrates. Just about every ailment is caused by excess inflammation in the body.

Even though I've been following a low-carb diet for many years, I still struggle with the underlying cause of my Graves' disease. I've also started to show signs of vitiligo, which is another autoimmune disease that causes white patches on the skin. A test done with a functional medicine doctor showed that I still have high immune activity as well. This is an indication that my immune system is mistakenly attacking healthy cells in my body, which is a sign of having one or more autoimmune diseases.

Consuming dairy and gluten in foods has been shown to be most inflammatory. All of my recipes are gluten-free, and because of the link between autoimmune disorders and dairy, I've been moving away from consuming dairy products, too. It's not difficult to replace heavy cream in keto recipes. That's easily done with coconut cream or using thickened almond milk, flax milk, or hemp milk. However, it's tough to find keto-friendly alternatives to cheese for many recipes, and that's where I've struggled the most in going dairy-free.

I experimented with the autoimmune protocol (AIP) diet and discovered that giving up dairy, as well as eliminating nuts and seeds, made me feel a whole lot better. (Unfortunately, coffee is a seed, so it had to go, too.) And I lost weight without even trying. I believe the reason is that removing problematic foods like dairy reduces inflammation in the body, and excess body fat is a sign of inflammation. If you find yourself struggling to lose fat, consider going beyond basic keto and start removing inflammatory foods to see which ones you are sensitive to.

How do you determine food sensitivities? There are blood tests, but they don't always tell the whole story. I took one and dairy wasn't on the list, even though eliminating certain dairy foods made me feel better. That's because the test I took only looked at IgG levels, which is just one of the many immune system response signals. An elimination diet is a much better (and cheaper) way to test for food sensitivities.

With an elimination diet, you'll remove a particular food like dairy for two to three weeks. Then, you'll see if a certain symptom like acne (common with dairy sensitivity), headaches, or bloating improves.

The AIP diet is a type of elimination diet. But rather than removing one food at a time, it removes the most common inflammatory foods and then slowly reintroduces them one at a time to see if certain symptoms return. I've included many AIP recipes in this cookbook since I feel the protocol is helpful for those with autoimmune conditions like me.

From my own experience with food-sensitivity testing at home, I discovered I'm sensitive to most low-carb sweeteners. Erythritol and fiber sweeteners result in gas and bloating for me. Stevia and monkfruit extracts are the ones I tolerate best. That's why I prefer them over all the others.

I encourage you to experiment with eliminating certain popular ketogenic foods (such as dairy and nuts) from your own diet to see if this helps with any inflammatory issues you are having. Also, if you haven't already given up gluten, you may want to start. It's one of the most inflammatory foods of all.

DAIRY ALTERNATIVES

Popular diets like Whole30 and paleo eliminate dairy for good reason. It's known to be one of the most inflammatory foods because most people are sensitive to dairy products and don't even know it. Humans were never meant to consume milk from another mammal. Heating cow's milk during pasteurization is another problem. It's done to kill any harmful pathogens and prevent milk from turning sour, but pasteurization also destroys some of the nutrients in milk and changes the structure of milk proteins.

I've found that it's fairly easy to replace cow's milk products in keto recipes. There's a wide variety of nut, seed, and coconut milk products that can be used in place of cow's milk. And you can even make your own! Eliminating dairy usually provides additional health benefits when used along with a keto diet. Therefore, I want to lay out some possible substitutes that may work if you're avoiding dairy.

BUTTER · My favorite swap for butter is to use butter-flavored coconut oil. The buttery flavor comes from fermented plants. It works well in baking and for frying. I've even used it in coffee and tea, but it's not the best to use for things like buttercream frosting as it can easily become liquid at room temperature. When coconut oil isn't an option, I've found that plant-based vegan butter works well. For recipes that use butter as a fat but in which the flavor of butter isn't necessary, coconut oil and lard make excellent substitutes.

I don't recommend using ghee in place of butter, even though most of the dairy proteins have been removed. It's still a dairy product and people with autoimmune disorders can still have a sensitivity to it.

HEAVY CREAM · For most recipes, heavy cream can be replaced with coconut cream. I look for brands that contain only coconut and water with no additives like guar gum. If you can't easily find it, canned coconut milk can be placed in the refrigerator overnight and then the solid part (which is the cream) can be separated out.

If you don't like coconut or have a reaction to it, a nut milk like unsweetened almond milk (see recipe, page 210) can be used instead, but it's a lot thinner than heavy cream, so a low-carb thickener like glucomannan may be needed.

YOGURT/SOUR CREAM · Yogurt and sour cream can be used interchangeably in recipes. I recommend using dairy-free yogurt in place of sour cream. If you have an electric pressure cooker with a yogurt-making function, you can follow my dairy-free yogurt recipe on LowCarbYum.com to make yogurt from coconut milk, nut milk, or seed milk.

Cheese

It can be nearly impossible when using nondairy cheeses to get that gooey stretchiness that makes cheesy recipes so appealing, and most dairy-free cheese doesn't melt as well as real cheese does. But it's possible to get some of the stretch and melting with cheese alternatives. Most of the commercially available dairy-free cheese products have a lot of added starch to give them a cheese-like texture, and if it's a grated nondairy cheese product, it may contain even more to keep the pieces from sticking to each other. Other products like almond milk cream cheese spreads also contain stabilizers like xanthan gum and guar gum, which typically aren't recommended for those with autoimmune conditions.

Since it's so difficult to get a decent keto-friendly dairy-free cheese, I just eliminate the cheese if it's not an essential ingredient or skip the recipe altogether. But if you're really craving cheese on a dairy-free keto diet plan, here are some options:

NUTRITIONAL YEAST · If I'm just trying to add a little cheesy flavor to the recipe, I sprinkle in some nutritional yeast powder or flakes. It's also an ingredient that can enhance the taste of low-carb and gluten-free breads.

NUT CHEESE · Cashews, almonds, macadamia, and walnuts are popular nuts used to make non-dairy cheese. To make cheese, you simply soak the raw nuts overnight and then process until smooth in a food processor. Nutritional yeast and lemon juice or vinegar are typically added for flavor. Herbs and spices can also enhance the taste. If desired, the mixture can be strained through cheesecloth and then baked to make a more solid cheese. You'll find my favorite almond cheese recipe in this book on page 72.

VEGETABLE CHEESE · Cauliflower and zucchini can also be used for making cheese substitutes. The process for making it is similar to nut cheese, but instead of soaking, the vegetables are steamed and then processed with nutritional yeast and lemon juice or vinegar along with herbs and spices. For sliced cheese versions, either gelatin or agar agar is used to make the cheese solid. There's a zucchini cheese recipe available on LowCarbYum .com if you want to give it a try.

Recommended Kitchen Tools

As you move away from packaged foods, you may want to invest in some kitchen tools that can make food preparation easier. I've listed some of my favorites below.

FOOD PROCESSOR · The grating blade on food processors is the most efficient way to grate cheese and vegetables. A lot of keto recipes call for grated cheese, but the pre-grated kind has added starch.

You'll want to grate your own cheese to avoid the added carbs. And making your own cauliflower rice is a cinch when you have a food processor.

SPIRALIZER · Zucchini noodles, aka zoodles, are one of the best alternatives to pasta. For an easy keto spaghetti, just make your own with zucchini and a spiralizer. You can also spiralize yellow squash, cucumbers, cabbage, and even bell peppers!

SMOOTHIE BLENDER · These small blenders are great for more than just smoothies. I use them to powder granular sweetener, too.

COFFEE GRINDER · For special nut and seed flours, I've found a coffee grinder works better than a blender or food processor. I use it to make my own sunflower seed flour and flax meal. Of course, you can also use it to grind coffee beans.

SLOW COOKER · If it's hard for you to find time to cook, you may want to prep slow cooker meals on off days or the evening before. Then, just put your meal in the pot before leaving in the morning to slow cook all day while you are at work or running errands.

ELECTRIC PRESSURE COOKER · Food cooks much faster under pressure, so you can use an electric pressure cooker to cook large cuts of meat and whole chickens much more quickly than roasting. Most also function as a slow cooker, electric pot, and yogurt maker. I like to use mine for making dairy-free yogurt out of coconut cream and almond milk.

KITCHEN SCALE · Volume measurements aren't very accurate, so I like to use weight measurements for things like low-carb flours and grated cheese. Knowing the weight of your ingredients helps to ensure the recipe comes out the same every time. It's also a good idea to weigh out your food portions to ensure that you aren't overeating when using keto for weight loss.

MILK FROTHER · I used to use a smoothie blender for making my keto coffee and tea to get the fat to blend in well. However, with a milk frother, it's simple to blend butter, MCT oil, or coconut oil into your coffee and tea right inside a tall mug.

CREAM WHIPPER · Have you ever looked at the ingredients in a can of whipped cream? Not only are there sugars added, but preservatives, too. I like to make my own whipped cream using a cream whipper because there's only heavy cream and a low-carb sweetener added. And it's great for making dairy-free whipped coconut cream, too!

MANDOLINE · It can take tons of time slicing and dicing vegetables, but having a mandoline gets it done in a fraction of the time.

SILICONE BAKING MATS AND PANS · Greasing pans doesn't always make things release well after baking. That's why I like to use silicone baking mats and sheet pans. Using them ensures that your cookies and cakes won't stick, and the mats are a great reusable alternative to parchment paper.

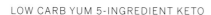

SAMPLE DAILY MEAL PLANS

Need some help figuring out what to eat each day? I put together seven examples of what a day of keto eating looks like. Just be sure that the calories, net carbs, and macros fit your individual needs. All of the examples are under 20 grams of net carbs a day.

DAY 1

Meal	Recipe	Calories	Carb	Fiber	Net Carb	Protein	Fat
Breakfast	Keto Coffee or Tea	151	1	0	1	0	17
	Bagel Thin	196	5	2	3	0	14
Lunch	Slow-Cooked Roasted Bone Broth	53	1	0	1	6	3
	Pesto Chicken Salad	405	3	1	2	16	36
Dinner	Wedge Salad	313	7	1	6	15	25
	Ginger Beef and Asparagus	231	3	1	2	26	12
Snack/Dessert	Nutty Crackers	151	4	2	2	4	13
	Total	**1,500**	**24**	**7**	**17**	**67**	**120**
	Daily Percentages				4.80%	18.93%	76.27%

DAY 2

Meal	Recipe	Calories	Carb	Fiber	Net Carb	Protein	Fat
Breakfast	Ginger-Turmeric Tea	6	1	0	1	0	0
	Bacon-Egg Cups	349	1	0	1	19	29
Lunch	Avocado Deviled Eggs	117	3	2	1	6	9
	Chicken Zoodle Soup	243	2	0	2	13	20
Dinner	Walnut Zucchini	143	4	1	2	2	13
	Quick "Breaded" Pork	346	6	3	3	28	23
Snack/Dessert	Crustless Baked Cheesecake	334	11	0	3	6	32
	Total	**1,538**	**28**	**6**	**13**	**74**	**126**
	Daily Percentages				3.51%	19.97%	76.52%

DAY 3

Meal	Recipe	Calories	Carb	Fiber	Net Carb	Protein	Fat
Breakfast	Keto Coffee or Tea	151	1	0	1	0	17
	Breakfast Burrito	287	6	3	3	11	24
Lunch	Salmon-Cucumber Salad	137	2	0	2	11	9
	Yellow Squash Soup	173	6	1	5	6	14
Dinner	Stir-Fried Squash and Pepper	89	5	1	2	1	7
	Garlic-Lemon Chicken	260	1	0	1	21	18
Snack/Dessert	Baked Coffee Custard	194	10	0	2	5	18
	Total	**1,291**	**31**	**5**	**16**	**55**	**107**
	Daily Percentages				5.13%	17.64%	77.23%

DAY 4

Meal	Recipe	Calories	Carb	Fiber	Net Carb	Protein	Fat
Breakfast	Keto Coffee or Tea	5	0	0	0	0	0
	Minute Muffin with Butter	270	4	2	2	5	26
	Breakfast Pizza	131	2	0	2	9	9
Lunch	Ground Beef and Cabbage	310	5	2	3	20	13
	Egg Drop Soup	105	1	0	1	3	9
Dinner	Almond Asparagus	206	8	4	4	5	18
	Roasted Chicken	319	1	0	1	27	21
Snack/Dessert	Chocolate Mousse	223	15	1	3	3	22
	Total	**1,569**	**36**	**9**	**16**	**72**	**118**
	Daily Percentages				4.53%	20.37%	75.11%

DAY 5

Meal	Recipe	Calories	Carb	Fiber	Net Carb	Protein	Fat
Breakfast	Green Tea Smoothie	171	10	7	3	2	14
Lunch	Sautéed Celery	70	1	0	1	0	7
	Crab Quiche	427	4	0	4	27	33
Dinner	Cauliflower Mash	119	7	2	5	4	8
	Beef Filet with Mushrooms	609	3	1	2	32	51
Snack/Dessert	Almond Butter Cookies	134	7	2	3	4	11
	Total	**1,530**	**32**	**12**	**18**	**69**	**124**
	Daily Percentages				4.92%	18.85%	76.23%

DAY 6

Meal	Recipe	Calories	Carb	Fiber	Net Carb	Protein	Fat
Breakfast	Keto Coffee or Tea	5	0	0	0	0	0
	Egg Casserole with Sausage and Spinach	349	1	0	1	18	29
	Egg Roll in a Bowl	225	5	1	4	14	16
Dinner	Creamed Spinach	211	5	2	2	7	19
	Baked Chicken Thighs	161	1	0	1	19	8
Snack/Dessert	No-Churn Vanilla Ice Cream	351	3	0	3	3	36
	Total	**1,302**	**15**	**3**	**11**	**61**	**108**
	Daily Percentages				3.49%	19.37%	77.14%

DAY 7

Meal	Recipe	Calories	Carb	Fiber	Net Carb	Protein	Fat
Breakfast	Keto Coffee or Tea	151	1	0	1	0	17
	Almond Flour Pancakes	189	6	3	3	3	17
Lunch	Seasoned Tortilla Chips	144	3	1	2	8	11
	Chicken Chili	243	3	1	2	37	8
Dinner	Roasted Broccoli	93	6	2	2	2	7
	Balsamic Halibut	224	0	0	0	28	11
Snack/Dessert	Vanilla Custard Pudding	428	3	0	3	6	43
	Total	**1,472**	**22**	**7**	**13**	**84**	**114**
	Daily Percentages				3.68%	23.76%	72.56%

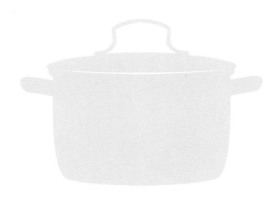

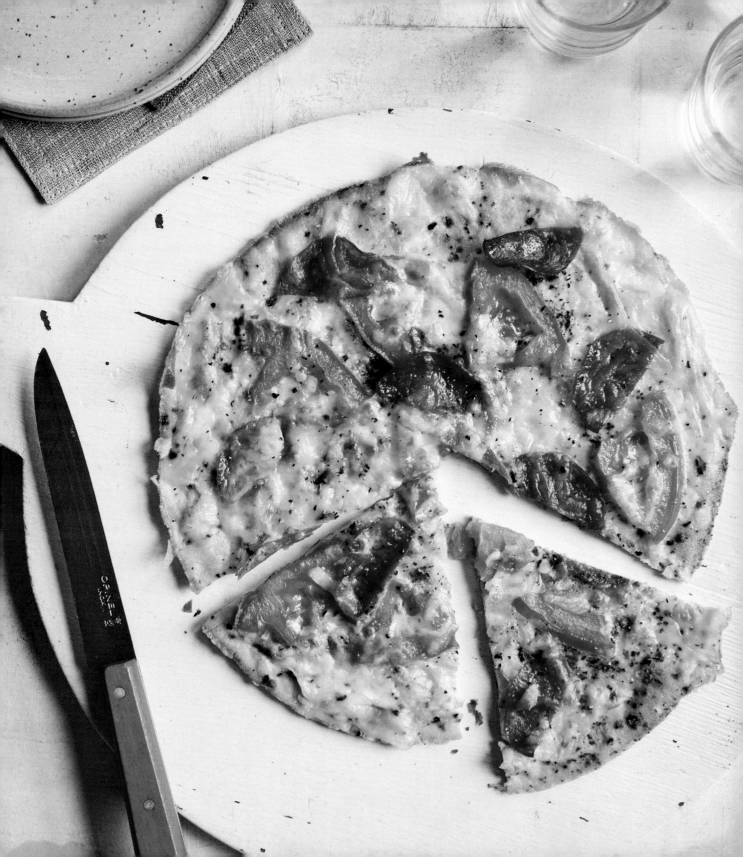

BREAKFAST

Almond Flour Pancakes 2

Scrambled Eggs with Crabmeat 4

Cauliflower "Mock" Porridge 5

Spinach-Tomato-Avocado Omelet 7

Granola Cereal 8

Bacon-Egg Cups 10

Minute Muffin 11

Coconut–Almond Butter Bars 13

Bagel Thins 14

Coconut Flour Waffles 17

Egg Casserole with Sausage and Spinach 18

Breakfast Burrito 20

Broccoli-Cheddar Egg Muffins 21

Breakfast Pizza 23

ALMOND FLOUR PANCAKES

PREP TIME: 10 minutes
COOK TIME: 5 minutes
TOTAL TIME: 15 minutes
SERVINGS: 8

DAIRY-FREE | PALEO

Fluffy, gluten-free pancakes with only 3 grams of net carbs in about 15 minutes. This was the breakfast recipe that got me hooked on the low-carb lifestyle. Regular pancakes never really satisfied me, but these almond flour ones will curb hunger for hours. Try serving them with my Maple Syrup (page 88).

2 cups blanched almond flour

4 large eggs

¼ cup oil (avocado oil or liquid coconut oil)

1 teaspoon baking soda

½ teaspoon salt

2 to 4 teaspoons monkfruit/erythritol granular sweetener (optional)

Heat a lightly oiled griddle to 350°F or a large skillet over medium-high heat.

In a medium bowl, combine the almond flour, eggs, oil, baking soda, salt, and sweetener, if using. Add ½ cup water and whisk briskly until well combined.

Pour about ⅓ cup of the pancake batter onto the hot griddle or skillet. Flip each one when the edges start to dry and the top is bubbling. Cook until browned on both sides. Remove the pancakes from the cooking surface to a rack or plate and repeat with the remaining batter.

NOTE

The eggs can be separated and the whites can be whipped and folded into the batter to create fluffier pancakes.

NUTRITIONAL DATA

189 calories, 17g fat, 399mg sodium, 3g fiber, 6g carbohydrates, 3g protein

3g net carbs, 7% carbs, 7% protein, 86% fat

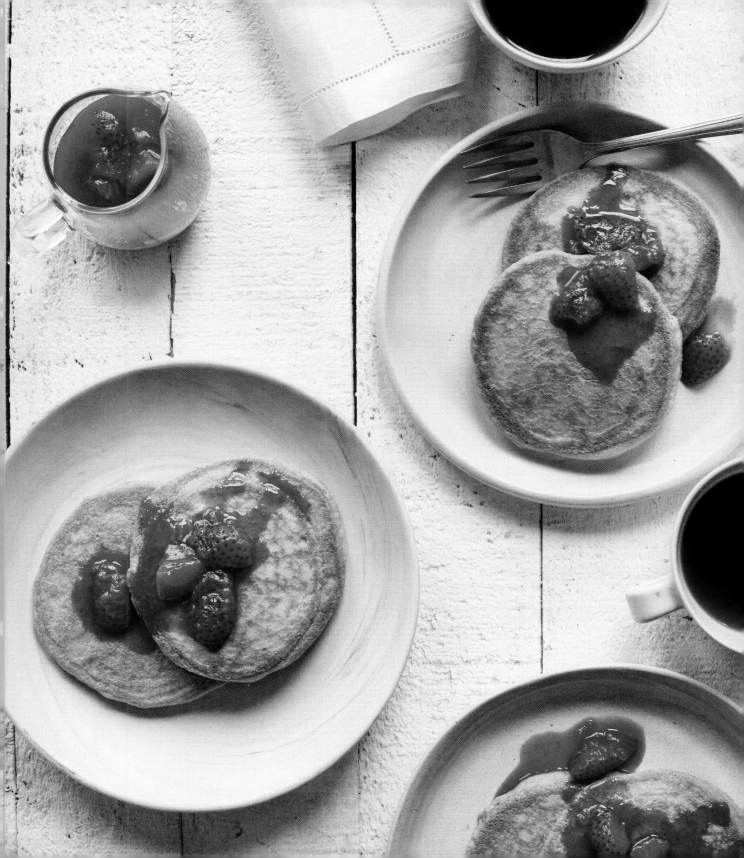

SCRAMBLED EGGS WITH CRABMEAT

PREP TIME: 2 minutes
COOK TIME: 7 minutes
TOTAL TIME: 9 minutes
SERVINGS: 4

NUT-FREE

Crab for breakfast? That's right, and I'm not even from Maryland! This combo of lump crabmeat, scrambled eggs, cheese, and chives is just as satisfying as lox and a bagel, but with zero carbs!

2 tablespoons butter

5 ounces canned crabmeat, drained

1 teaspoon chopped fresh chives

8 large eggs

½ cup grated cheddar cheese

Salt and black pepper

Melt the butter in a medium nonstick skillet over low heat. Add the crabmeat and chives and cook, stirring, for 2 minutes.

In a medium bowl, beat the eggs, then stir in the cheese. Pour the egg mixture over the crabmeat in the pan. Cook, stirring, until the eggs are cooked, about 3 minutes. Season with salt and pepper to taste.

NOTES

Other shellfish meat like lobster or scallops works well in place of the crab. Swiss cheese is also a great replacement for the cheddar cheese.

NUTRITIONAL DATA

161 calories, 9g fat, 402mg sodium, 0g fiber, 0g carbohydrates, 20g protein

0g net carbs, 0% carbs, 50% protein, 50% fat

CAULIFLOWER "MOCK" PORRIDGE

PREP TIME: 5 minutes
COOK TIME: 15 minutes
TOTAL TIME: 20 minutes
SERVINGS: 1

DAIRY-FREE | EGG-FREE | PALEO

Even Goldilocks would agree that this cauliflower porridge is "just right." It's got the same starchy, comfort-food texture as regular oats, but with a lot fewer carbs.

4 ounces cauliflower florets

½ cup Almond Milk (page 210) or other low-carb milk

⅛ teaspoon ground cinnamon

1 to 2 teaspoons monkfruit/erythritol granular sweetener

Sliced strawberries or other berries (optional)

Place the cauliflower and almond milk in a small pot. Bring to a boil over medium-high heat. Reduce the heat to medium-low, cover, and cook for 7 to 10 minutes until the cauliflower is fork-tender.

Remove from the heat. Let cool briefly and puree in a blender with the cinnamon and sweetener. Serve warm with berries on top, if desired.

NOTES

Add a dash of vanilla for extra flavor.

Great served with a Keto Coffee (page 210) for added fat.

NUTRITIONAL DATA

46 calories, 1g fat, 196mg sodium, 2g fiber, 11g carbohydrates, 5g erythritol, 2g protein

4g net carbs, 49% carbs, 24% protein, 27% fat

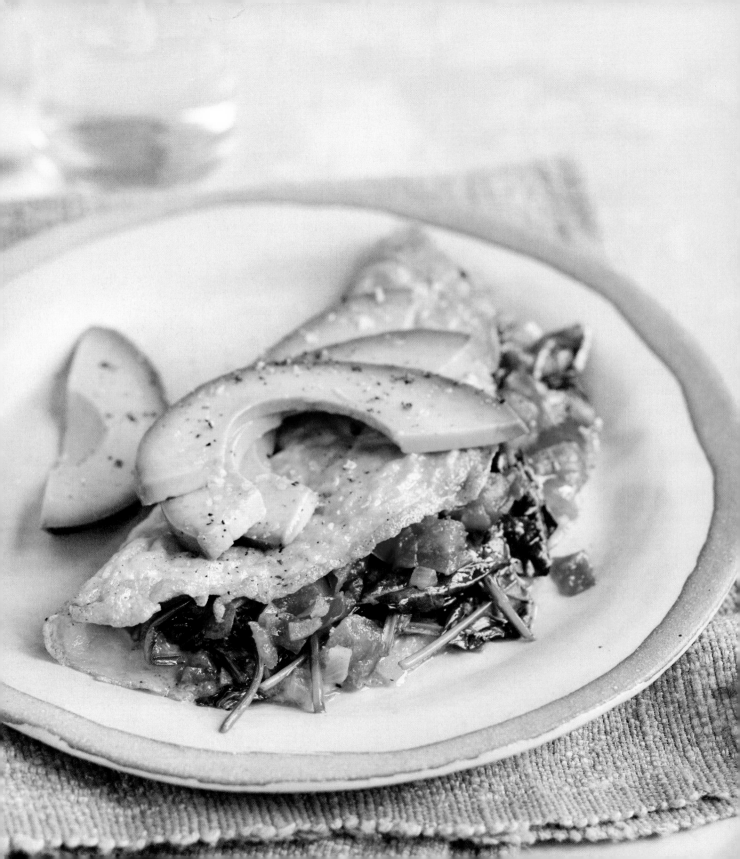

SPINACH-TOMATO-AVOCADO OMELET

PREP TIME: 5 minutes
COOK TIME: 10 minutes
TOTAL TIME: 15 minutes
SERVINGS: 1

DAIRY-FREE | NUT-FREE | PALEO

The biggest key to keto success is filling up with high-fat meals. When you start the day with an omelet loaded with healthy fat, you won't need a morning snack and may not even be hungry at lunchtime.

1 tablespoon extra-virgin olive oil

1 tablespoon chopped onion

1½ cups (1 ounce) baby spinach

¼ medium tomato, chopped

Salt and black pepper

2 large eggs, beaten

½ ripe avocado, sliced

Heat the olive oil in an 8-inch omelet pan over medium-high heat. Add the onion and cook, stirring, until translucent, about 5 minutes. Add the spinach and tomato and season to taste with the salt and black pepper. Cook, stirring, to wilt the spinach, 2 to 3 minutes, then remove from the pan to a plate.

In the same pan over low heat, add the beaten eggs, cover, and cook for 30 seconds. Add the sautéed spinach and tomato on one side of the omelet. Fold the omelet in half over itself, resembling a half-moon. Cook until the egg is set, 1 to 2 minutes more.

Serve immediately with the avocado slices on top.

NOTE

Add chopped bacon for extra flavor and fat.

NUTRITIONAL DATA

426 calories, 37g fat, 156mg sodium, 7g fiber, 12g carbohydrates, 14g protein

5g net carbs, 5% carbs, 14% protein, 81% fat

GRANOLA CEREAL

DAIRY-FREE | PALEO

PREP TIME: 10 minutes
COOK TIME: 16 minutes
TOTAL TIME: 26 minutes
SERVINGS: 8

Whether it's to fuel a long hike or just provide an energy boost in the morning for a normal workday, this homemade granola satisfies without unnecessary carbs and sugar. Serve about ⅓ cup per serving with low-carb milk or sprinkle on plain Greek-style yogurt.

1½ cups sliced almonds

1 cup pecans or walnuts

1 cup flaked unsweetened coconut

¼ cup coconut oil

2 large egg whites

Preheat the oven to 375°F. Line a sheet pan with parchment paper or a silicone baking mat.

Add the almonds, pecans, coconut, and coconut oil to a food processor. Pulse 20 times or to desired texture for granola. Stir in the egg whites.

Spread the mixture in an even layer on the lined sheet pan. Bake for 14 to 16 minutes until fragrant and crisp.

Allow to cool and then break into bite-size pieces. Store in an airtight container at room temperature for up to a week. For longer storage, refrigerate the granola.

NOTES

The coconut adds sweetness without sugar. However, those who prefer a sweeter cereal will want to add in sweetener and/or vanilla to taste. A teaspoon or two of cinnamon can also be added for enhanced flavor.

Other nuts and seeds can be substituted as well.

NUTRITIONAL DATA

334 calories, 32g fat, 16mg sodium, 5g fiber, 8g carbohydrates, 6g protein

3g net carbs, 4% carbs, 7% protein, 89% fat

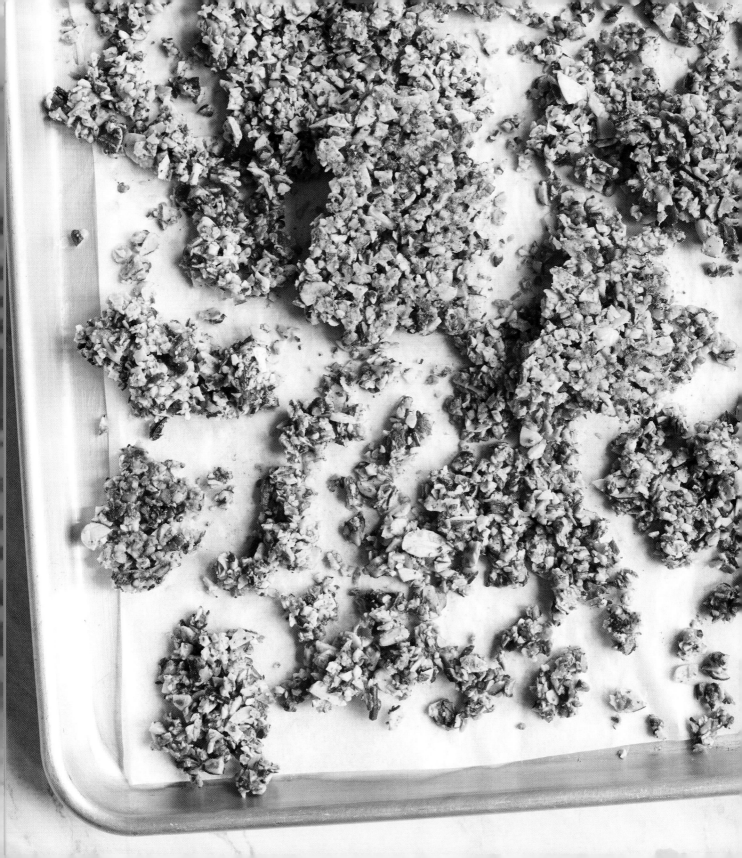

BACON-EGG CUPS

NUT-FREE

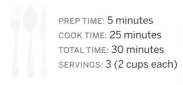

PREP TIME: 5 minutes
COOK TIME: 25 minutes
TOTAL TIME: 30 minutes
SERVINGS: 3 (2 cups each)

Pressed for time in the morning? Take a classic bacon and eggs recipe, prepare in muffin tins and voilà! An instant high-protein, high-fat healthy fast-food breakfast that you can reheat in the microwave or toaster oven.

6 slices bacon, partially cooked and still bendable

1½ cups (1 ounce) baby spinach

1 ounce grated cheese (Swiss, cheddar, and Parmesan are good choices)

6 large eggs

Salt and black pepper

3 fresh chives, chopped

1 teaspoon chopped fresh parsley (optional)

Preheat the oven to 400°F. Grease 6 muffin cups or line with silicone liners.

Line the sides and bottom of each muffin cup with a slice of bacon to form a cup. Divide the spinach and cheese evenly among the bacon cups. Crack each egg into a bowl and gently pour one egg over the spinach and cheese in each cup.

Season the top of each egg with salt and black pepper and then sprinkle the chives and parsley (if using) on top.

Bake for 20 to 25 minutes, until the bacon is fully cooked and the eggs no longer jiggle.

NOTE

The eggs can be beaten first for a more frittata-style muffin.

NUTRITIONAL DATA

349 calories, 29g fat, 482mg sodium, 0g fiber, 1g carbohydrates, 19g protein

1g net carbs, 1% carbs, 22% protein, 77% fat

MINUTE MUFFIN

DAIRY-FREE

PREP TIME: 3 minutes
COOK TIME: 2 minutes
TOTAL TIME: 5 minutes
SERVINGS: 2

High-protein almond flour and healthy coconut flour team up as the perfect, satiating combo for this health muffin that takes two minutes to cook. You can toast it and serve it with fried eggs, or use it to make a bacon-and-egg sandwich to go.

3 tablespoons blanched almond flour

1 tablespoon coconut flour

½ teaspoon baking powder

⅛ teaspoon salt

1 large egg

1 tablespoon avocado oil

Combine the almond flour, coconut flour, baking powder, and salt in a microwavable coffee mug or ramekin. Add the egg and avocado oil and stir well with a fork.

Microwave on high for 1 to 1½ minutes, until set.

Remove the muffin from the mug using a butter knife to release the sides, then flip it onto a plate. Slice the muffin in half for two servings. It can be sliced again into two thinner rounds to use for a sandwich.

NOTE

The muffins are excellent toasted and served with butter or butter-flavored coconut oil.

NUTRITIONAL DATA

168 calories, 14g fat, 184mg sodium, 2g fiber, 4g carbohydrates, 5g protein

2g net carbs, 5% carbs, 13% protein, 82% fat

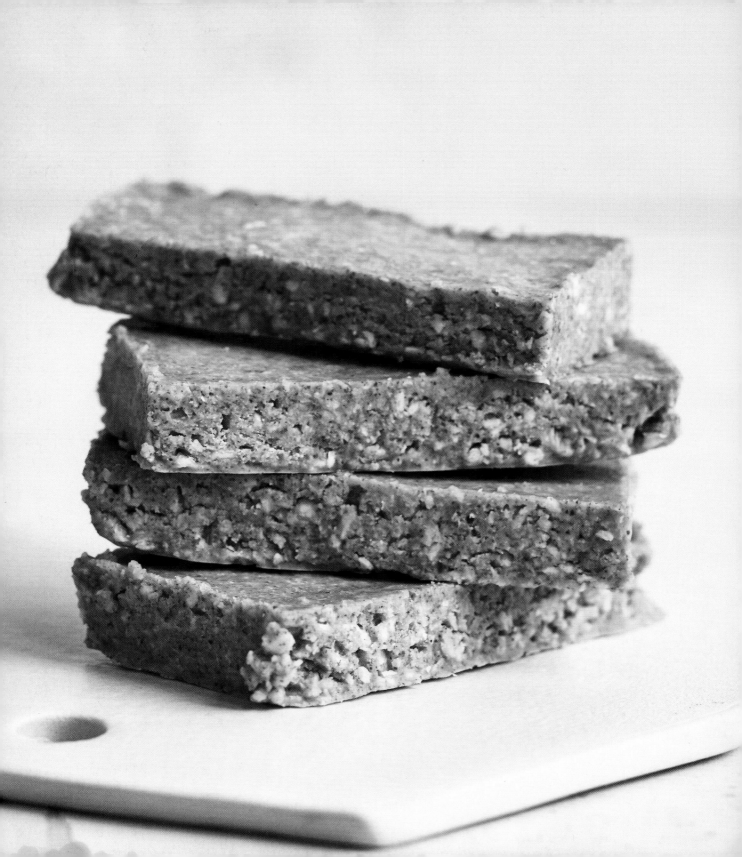

COCONUT–ALMOND BUTTER BARS

DAIRY-FREE | EGG-FREE

PREP TIME: 5 minutes
COOK TIME: 25 minutes
TOTAL TIME: 30 minutes
SERVINGS: 8

Most commercially sold breakfast bars fail in their function as meal replacements. Because of the sugar and lack of healthy fats, they leave you hungry soon after eating them. By making your own keto bars, you get all the convenience and nutrition without the insulin spike.

¾ cup unsweetened almond butter

¾ cup unsweetened shredded coconut

¼ cup coconut oil, melted

2 tablespoons monkfruit/erythritol granular sweetener

Line an 8 × 8-inch baking pan with parchment paper.

Combine the almond butter, shredded coconut, coconut oil, and sweetener in a large bowl. Spread the mixture into the prepared pan.

Refrigerate or freeze until solid. Slice into 8 bars.

NOTES

The coconut can be replaced with nuts or low-carb chocolate chips to change things up.

The bars will get soft at room temperature so they should be eaten chilled from the freezer or refrigerator.

NUTRITIONAL DATA

327 calories, 32g fat, 12mg sodium, 3g fiber, 10g carbohydrates, 4g erythritol, 6g protein

3g net carbs, 4% carbs, 7% protein, 89% fat

BAGEL THINS

NUT-FREE

PREP TIME: 10 minutes
COOK TIME: 18 minutes
TOTAL TIME: 28 minutes
SERVINGS: 8

Love losing weight on keto but desperately miss bagels? Say hello to eating bagels again. The blend of mozzarella and cream cheese makes the texture of these gluten-free bagels similar to the real thing. They freeze well so be sure to make extra for later!

60 grams coconut flour (about ½ cup)

2 teaspoons baking powder, preferably aluminum-free

250 grams shredded mozzarella cheese (about 2½ cups)

110 grams cream cheese (about 4 ounces)

3 large eggs, beaten (at room temperature)

Preheat the oven to 400°F. Line a baking sheet with parchment paper.

Mix the coconut flour and baking powder in a small bowl. Set aside.

In a microwave oven, melt the mozzarella cheese and cream cheese in a bowl on high power for 1 minute. Stir. Microwave on high for another minute. Stir again.

Using your hands, mix the beaten eggs and coconut flour mixture into the cheeses until a well-blended dough is formed. The dough should be a bit sticky.

Divide the dough into 8 pieces and roll out each piece into a rope, then connect the ends to form a bagel shape. The dough is easier to work with if your hands are wet.

Place the bagels on the parchment paper–lined baking sheet. Bake for 12 to 16 minutes, until browned. Transfer the bagels to a rack to cool completely.

NOTES

Adding a tablespoon of almond flour gives a more bread-like texture, while a tablespoon of nutritional yeast can enhance the flavor.

Seasonings like garlic and onion powder can be added if desired. A couple tablespoons of melted butter can be added to the dough for a buttery flavor.

Toasted sesame seeds or an everything bagel seasoning blend can be sprinkled on top before baking.

It's best to weigh the ingredients on a kitchen scale for better accuracy.

Place eggs in warm water for 10 to 15 minutes to bring them to room temperature quickly.

NUTRITIONAL DATA

196 calories, 14g fat, 552mg sodium, 2g fiber, 5g carbohydrates, 10g protein

6g net carbs, 7% carbs, 22% protein, 71% fat

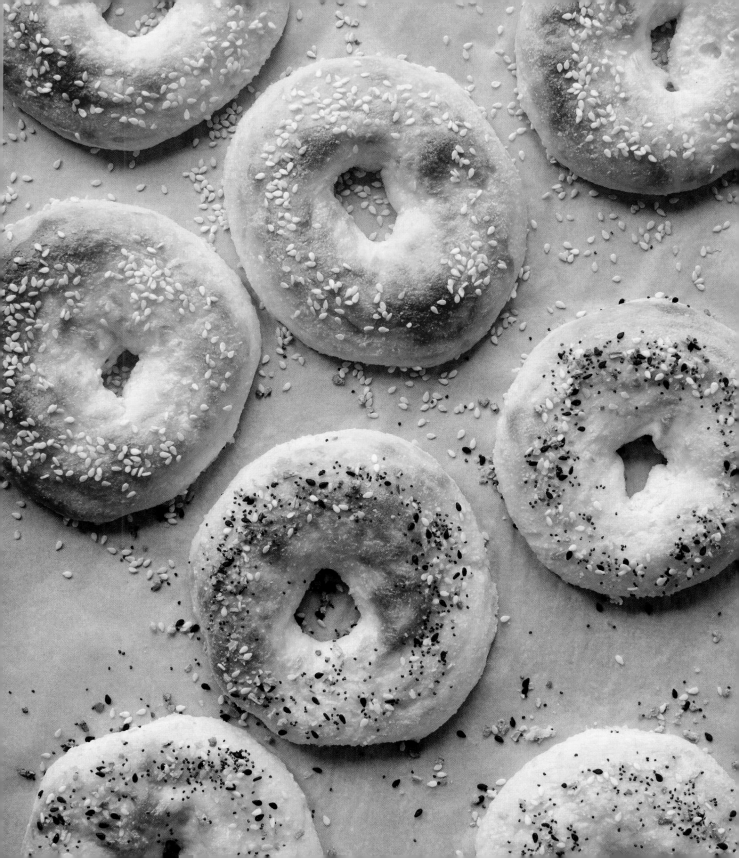

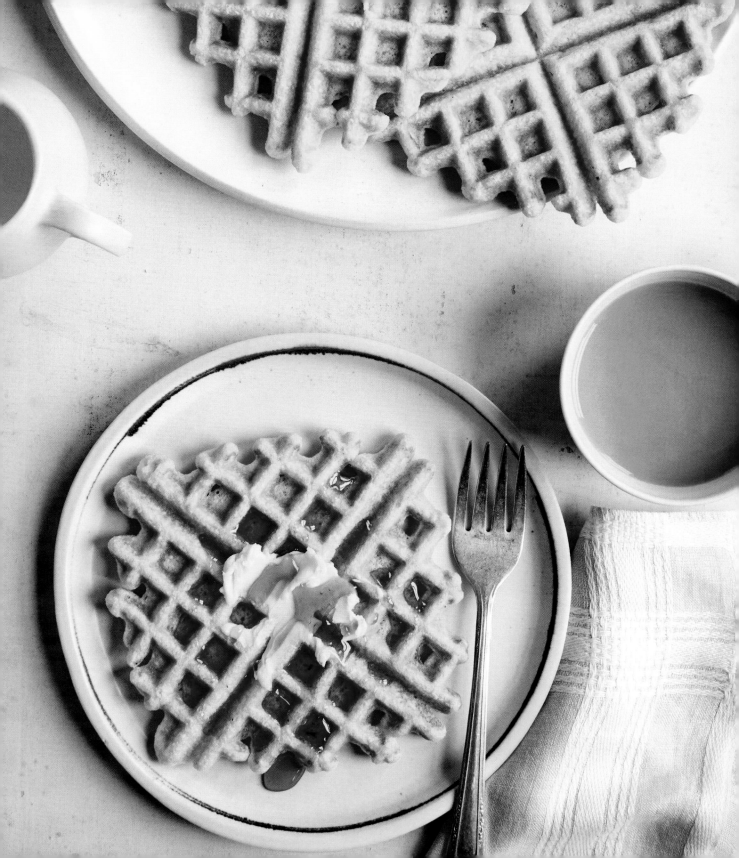

COCONUT FLOUR WAFFLES

NUT-FREE

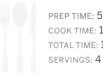

PREP TIME: 5 minutes
COOK TIME: 10 minutes
TOTAL TIME: 15 minutes
SERVINGS: 4

Coconut flour is the secret to making light and fluffy keto waffles, and they are perfect for making big batches at once and freezing single servings for later. Just pop the frozen waffles in the toaster or microwave! Try serving them with my Maple Syrup (page 88).

4 tablespoons butter or ghee, melted

5 large eggs

2 teaspoons monkfruit/erythritol granular sweetener (optional)

½ teaspoon salt

½ teaspoon baking powder

⅓ cup coconut flour

In a blender or in a mixing bowl using an electric mixer, mix the butter and eggs until combined thoroughly. Add the sweetener, salt, and baking powder and mix to combine. Mix in the coconut flour until completely combined without any lumps. Let the batter sit for a few minutes to thicken. If needed, a little water can be added to thin the batter.

Pour the batter into a waffle maker and cook according to the waffle maker's directions. Typically, the waffles are done when the steaming stops or slows down.

NOTES

Coconut oil may be used in place of the butter or ghee.

A hand whisk should work to blend the ingredients together.

NUTRITIONAL DATA

221 calories, 17g fat, 490mg sodium, 3g fiber, 8g carbohydrates, 2g erythritol, 8g protein

3g net carbs, 10% carbs, 16% protein, 74% fat

EGG CASSEROLE WITH SAUSAGE AND SPINACH

NUT-FREE

PREP TIME: 5 minutes
COOK TIME: 40 minutes
TOTAL TIME: 45 minutes
SERVINGS: 9

Weekend food prep always includes casseroles to last the workweek. This easy breakfast casserole should provide you with several keto-friendly meals to enjoy for breakfast or lunch. It can be frozen for later too!

1 tablespoon extra-virgin olive oil

7½ cups (5 ounces) baby spinach

1 pound bulk sausage meat

6 large eggs

1 cup coconut milk or Almond Milk (page 210)

⅛ teaspoon salt

Dash black pepper

2 cups shredded cheddar cheese

Preheat the oven to 350°F. Grease an 8 × 8-inch baking pan.

Heat the oil in a skillet over medium heat. Add the spinach and cook, stirring frequently, until wilted, about 1 minute. Transfer to a plate.

Add the sausage to the same skillet and cook, stirring and breaking up the meat, until browned. Remove from the heat.

In a bowl, beat together the eggs and coconut milk. Season with the salt and black pepper. Pour a thin layer of the egg mixture into the prepared pan. Cover with the sausage and spinach. Sprinkle on the shredded cheese. Pour the rest of the egg mixture evenly over the top.

Bake for 20 to 25 minutes, until lightly brown on top.

NOTES

The sausage can be replaced with ham or bacon, and other cheese blends can be used to change the flavor.

Freeze in single servings for easy meals later.

NUTRITIONAL DATA

349 calories, 29g fat, 533mg sodium, 0g fiber, 1g carbohydrates, 18g protein

1g net carbs, 1% carbs, 21% protein, 77% fat

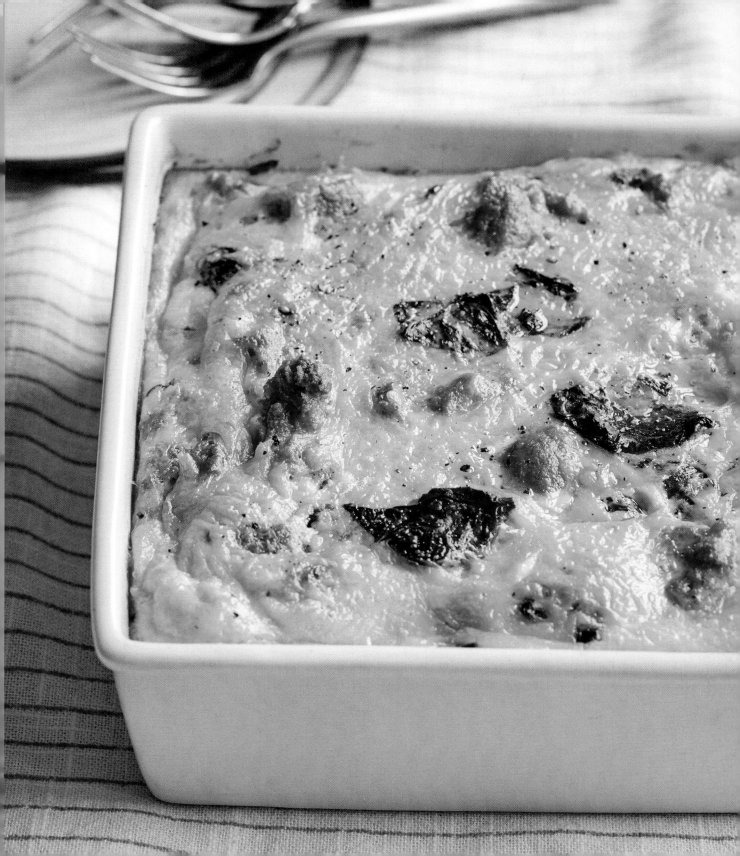

BREAKFAST BURRITO

DAIRY-FREE | NUT-FREE | PALEO

PREP TIME: 10 minutes
COOK TIME: 10 minutes
TOTAL TIME: 20 minutes
SERVINGS: 2

Cabbage leaves are an ultra-low-carb alternative for flour tortillas when making breakfast burritos. Just fill them with scrambled eggs and your favorite keto-friendly add-ins like bacon and avocado.

2 cabbage leaves

3 slices bacon, cooked

2 large eggs, beaten

½ avocado, diced

2 tablespoons diced tomato

Wash and dry the cabbage leaves.

Cook the bacon in a skillet over medium heat until crispy. Set aside on a plate, reserving the bacon grease in the skillet. Scramble the eggs in the bacon grease in the skillet.

Chop the bacon when cooled a bit. On top of the cabbage leaves, divide the bacon, scrambled eggs, avocado, and tomato. Roll up each leaf around the fillings like a burrito and serve.

NOTE

Lettuce can be used, but cabbage leaves tend to hold up better.

NUTRITIONAL DATA

287 calories, 24g fat, 308mg sodium, 3g fiber, 6g carbohydrates, 11g protein

3g net carbs, 4% carbs, 16% protein, 79% fat

BROCCOLI-CHEDDAR EGG MUFFINS

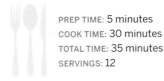

PREP TIME: 5 minutes
COOK TIME: 30 minutes
TOTAL TIME: 35 minutes
SERVINGS: 12

NUT-FREE

Egg muffins are a fantastic portable breakfast. It's another filling dish
I created for those 14-hour workdays I used to slog through. Two of these would keep
me going until midday without thinking about food.

10 ounces broccoli florets

8 large eggs

¾ cup heavy cream

1½ cups grated cheddar cheese

½ teaspoon salt

½ teaspoon onion powder

⅛ teaspoon black pepper

Preheat the oven to 375°F. Grease a 12-cup muffin pan or line the cups with silicone liners.

Steam the broccoli until crisp-tender, 4 to 5 minutes.

In large bowl, beat the eggs with the heavy cream. Stir in the broccoli, cheese, salt, onion powder, and black pepper.

Divide the mixture evenly among the prepared muffin cups. Bake for 20 to 25 minutes, until the tops begin to brown.

NOTES

The mixture can also be poured into a 9½-inch deep-dish pie pan and baked for 30 to 40 minutes for a crustless quiche.

NUTRITIONAL DATA

158 calories, 13g fat, 239mg sodium, 0g fiber, 2g carbohydrates, 8g protein

2g net carbs, 5% carbs, 20% protein, 75% fat

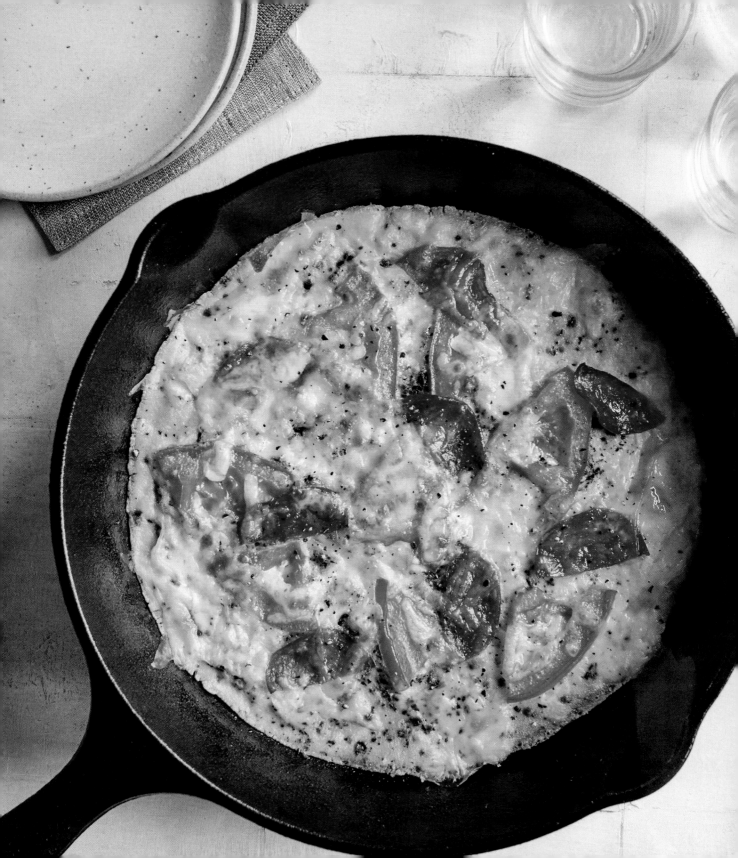

BREAKFAST PIZZA

NUT-FREE

PREP TIME: 5 minutes
COOK TIME: 10 minutes
TOTAL TIME: 15 minutes
SERVINGS: 1

Pizza for breakfast? Why not, especially when there's only 2 grams of net carbs in the whole thing? One of my all-time favorite discoveries of low-carb cooking was that eggs make an excellent crust for all your favorite pizza toppings.

2 large eggs, beaten well

Dash Italian seasoning

Salt and black pepper

2 slices tomato, quartered

4 slices pepperoni, cut in half

1 ounce mozzarella cheese, grated

Grease an oven-safe 8-inch round high-sided skillet (a seasoned cast-iron pan is perfect). Heat the prepared pan over medium heat. Set an oven rack 6 inches under the broiler and preheat the broiler.

Pour the eggs into the hot pan, then sprinkle on the Italian seasoning and season with salt and black pepper.

When the eggs have started to set on the bottom, top with the tomato slices, pepperoni, and mozzarella. Cover the pan and cook for 1 to 2 minutes to fully cook the eggs. Remove from the heat.

Place the pan under the broiler for 1 to 2 minutes to lightly brown the cheese.

NOTES

Other pizza toppings can be added as well, like cooked sausage, mushrooms, or spinach.

NUTRITIONAL DATA

131 calories, 9g fat, 223mg sodium, 0g fiber, 2g carbohydrates, 9g protein

2g net carbs, 6% carbs, 29% protein, 65% fat

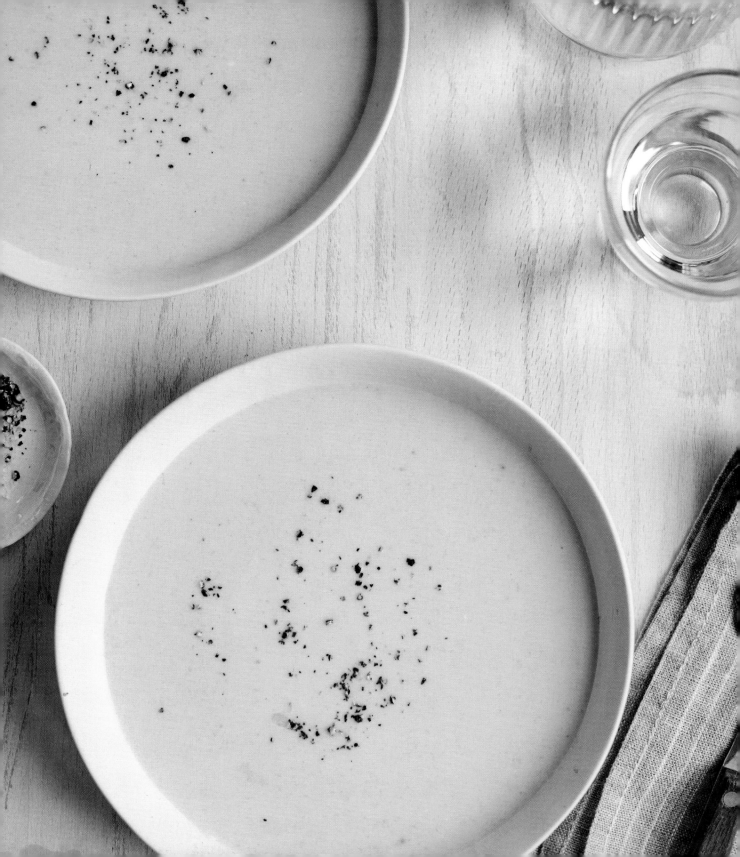

SOUPS AND STEWS

Slow-Cooked Roasted Bone Broth 26

Broccoli-Cheese Soup 27

Sausage-Kale Soup 28

Chicken Zoodle Soup 31

Egg Drop Soup 32

Oyster Stew 34

No-Bean Chili 35

Creamy Avocado Soup 37

Cabbage and Ground Beef Soup 38

Cream of Mushroom Soup 40

Pumpkin Soup 41

Yellow Squash Soup 43

Roasted Brussels with Bacon Soup 44

Chicken Chili 47

SLOW-COOKED ROASTED BONE BROTH

DAIRY-FREE | NUT-FREE | EGG-FREE | PALEO, AIP

PREP TIME: 10 minutes
COOK TIME: 48 hours
TOTAL TIME: 48 hours 10 minutes
SERVINGS: 8

Our ancestors made bone broth out of necessity, but today bone broth is enjoying a resurgence because of its known health benefits. In addition to its robust flavor, it contains collagen protein, which is good for your immune system, digestion, skin, hair, and nails.

1 carcass and pan drippings from a whole roasted chicken

2 cloves garlic

2 tablespoons apple cider vinegar

2 to 3 cups vegetable scraps (celery works well)

1 teaspoon sea salt

Add enough water to the roasted chicken pan drippings to make 8 cups of liquid total. Heat the pan if necessary to free the browned bits. Pour the liquid into a slow cooker and add the chicken carcass, garlic, vinegar, vegetable scraps, and salt. Cook on low for 24 to 48 hours. Longer cooking times will allow more of the nutrients to come out of the bones as well as provide a more robust flavor.

Strain the broth, discarding the solids, and transfer it to mason jars or other heat-safe glass containers. Store in the refrigerator for up to 3 or 4 days.

The broth can also be frozen for longer storage, up to 6 months.

NOTES

The cooking time can be reduced by using an electric (or traditional) pressure cooker: pressure cook on high for 3 to 4 hours first and then slow cook for 8 to 10 hours.

If using other animal bones like beef or venison, the bones should be roasted until brown first. And for the best flavor, be sure to have a little meat on the bones.

NUTRITIONAL DATA

53 calories, 3g fat, 296mg sodium, 0g fiber, 1g carbohydrates, 6g protein

1g net carbs, 7% carbs, 44% protein, 49% fat

BROCCOLI-CHEESE SOUP

PREP TIME: 10 minutes
COOK TIME: 20 minutes
TOTAL TIME: 30 minutes
SERVINGS: 8

NUT-FREE | EGG-FREE

This soup is probably one reason I've had trouble going completely dairy-free—I just love cheddar and broccoli together because they are such a great flavor combination. This rich, thick, and creamy soup can be enjoyed any time of year.

1½ pounds chopped broccoli (about 3 cups)

4 cups Slow-Cooked Roasted Bone Broth (page 26)

1 cup heavy cream

4 ounces cream cheese

8 ounces mild cheddar cheese, shredded

Salt and black pepper

Steam the broccoli until crisp-tender, about 5 minutes.

Add the broccoli, broth, heavy cream, and cream cheese to a food processor or high-speed blender and blend until smooth. Transfer the mixture to a pot, bring to a low boil over high heat, then immediately reduce the heat and simmer for about 10 minutes more. Stir in the cheddar cheese until melted, about 5 minutes. Season to taste with salt and black pepper.

NOTES

If the soup is too thick, a little water can be added to thin it.

NUTRITIONAL DATA

300 calories, 25g fat, 786mg sodium, 2g fiber, 7g carbohydrates, 11g protein

5g net carbs, 7% carbs, 15% protein, 78% fat

SAUSAGE-KALE SOUP

DAIRY-FREE | NUT-FREE | EGG-FREE | PALEO

PREP TIME: 10 minutes
COOK TIME: 1 hour, 20 minutes
TOTAL TIME: 1½ hours
SERVINGS: 6

Hearty enough for a light meal or great for a comforting, heartwarming appetizer. I use chicken bone broth as the base. It's a double dose of filling protein and nutrient-rich veggies.

1 pound ground sausage

8 ounces sliced white mushrooms

2 cloves garlic, minced

4 cups Slow-Cooked Roasted Bone Broth (page 26)

8 ounces kale, cut into bite-size pieces

Salt and black pepper

In a Dutch oven or large pot over medium-high heat, add the sausage and cook, stirring and breaking up the meat with a wooden spoon, until browned, about 10 minutes. Add the mushrooms and garlic and cook, stirring, for another 2 to 3 minutes. Pour in the chicken broth along with 4 cups water and bring to a boil over medium-high heat.

Add the kale and season to taste with salt and black pepper. Reduce the heat to low and simmer, covered, for about an hour. Adjust the seasonings if needed.

NOTES

The mushrooms can be replaced with sliced radishes, if desired.

This one can be AIP-friendly, too, by using homemade sausage meat or just plain ground beef and eliminating the pepper.

NUTRITIONAL DATA

265 calories, 20g fat, 995mg sodium, 0g fiber, 5g carbohydrates, 14g protein

5g net carbs, 8% carbs, 22% protein, 70% fat

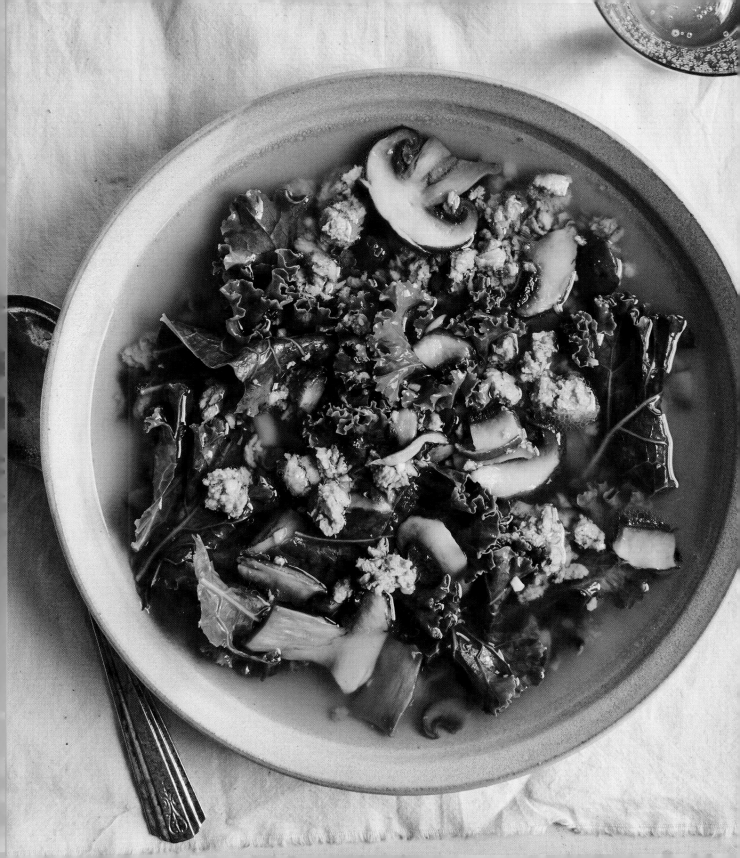

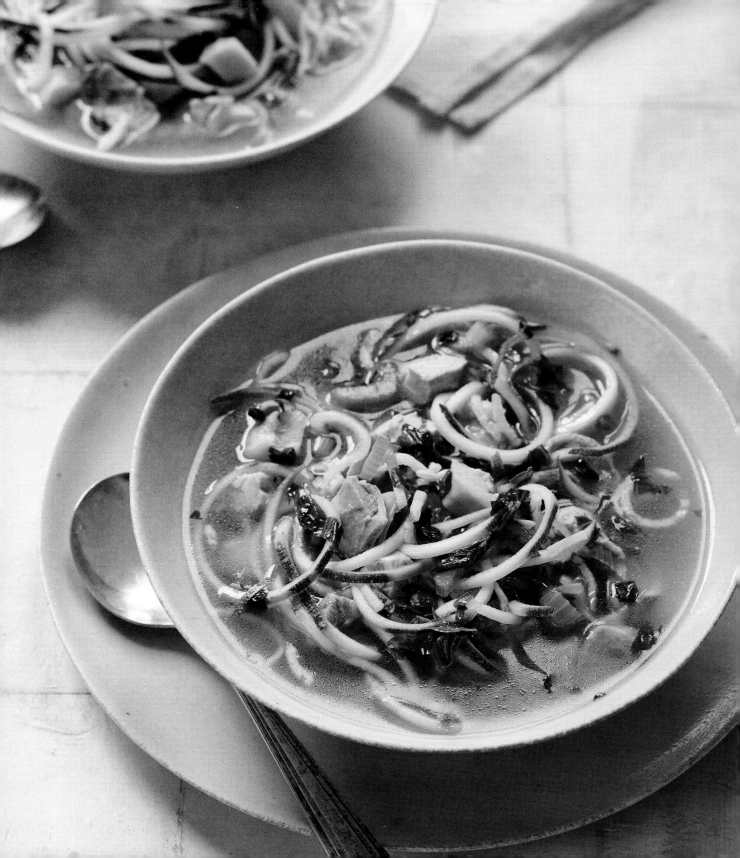

CHICKEN ZOODLE SOUP

PREP TIME: 10 minutes
COOK TIME: 30 minutes
TOTAL TIME: 40 minutes
SERVINGS: 4

DAIRY-FREE | NUT-FREE | EGG-FREE | PALEO, AIP

Noodles in broth have been served to the sick for centuries, but you don't need to be ill to enjoy chicken noodle soup. It's actually the chicken broth that does a body good, not the wheat! With spiralized zucchini serving as the noodles, you can enjoy this medicinal soup on keto.

2 tablespoons coconut oil

4 stalks celery

4 cups Slow-Cooked Roasted Bone Broth (page 26)

2 cups cubed cooked boneless chicken thighs

2 teaspoons chopped fresh basil

1 medium zucchini, spiralized

¼ teaspoon salt

Fresh parsley (optional), for garnish

NOTES

Add a small turnip or radish, peeled and diced, for mock potatoes.

NUTRITIONAL DATA

243 calories, 20g fat, 982mg sodium, 0g fiber, 2g carbohydrates, 13g protein

2g net carbs, 3% carbs, 22% protein, 75% fat

Heat the oil in a pot over medium heat. Add the celery and cook, stirring, for about 10 minutes. Add the broth, chicken, and basil and bring to a boil over high heat. Reduce the heat, cover, and simmer for about 20 minutes. Remove from the heat.

Stir in the zucchini and cover the pot for about 10 minutes to let the zucchini soften before serving.

EGG DROP SOUP

DAIRY-FREE | **NUT-FREE** | **PALEO**

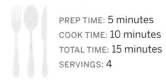

PREP TIME: 5 minutes
COOK TIME: 10 minutes
TOTAL TIME: 15 minutes
SERVINGS: 4

I used to love sipping egg drop soup when we'd go to our favorite Chinese restaurant. These days, I'm making it at home, but without a high-carb thickener like cornstarch. Same great flavor with only 1 net gram of carbohydrates!

2 tablespoons coconut oil

2 cloves garlic, minced

4 cups Slow-Cooked Roasted Bone Broth (page 26)

1 teaspoon minced fresh ginger

2 large eggs, beaten

Pinch red pepper flakes

Salt and black pepper

Heat the coconut oil in a pot over medium heat. Add the garlic and cook, stirring, until fragrant, about 3 minutes. Add the broth and ginger and bring to a boil over high heat. Reduce the heat to low, then, while whisking, slowly pour in the beaten eggs. Add the red pepper flakes and season to taste with salt and black pepper.

Remove from the heat and serve.

NOTES

Splash in some coconut aminos or tamari along with a sprinkling of chopped green onions for extra flavor.

NUTRITIONAL DATA

105 calories, 9g fat, 861mg sodium, 0g fiber, 1g carbohydrates, 3g protein

1g net carbs, 4% carbs, 12% protein, 84% fat

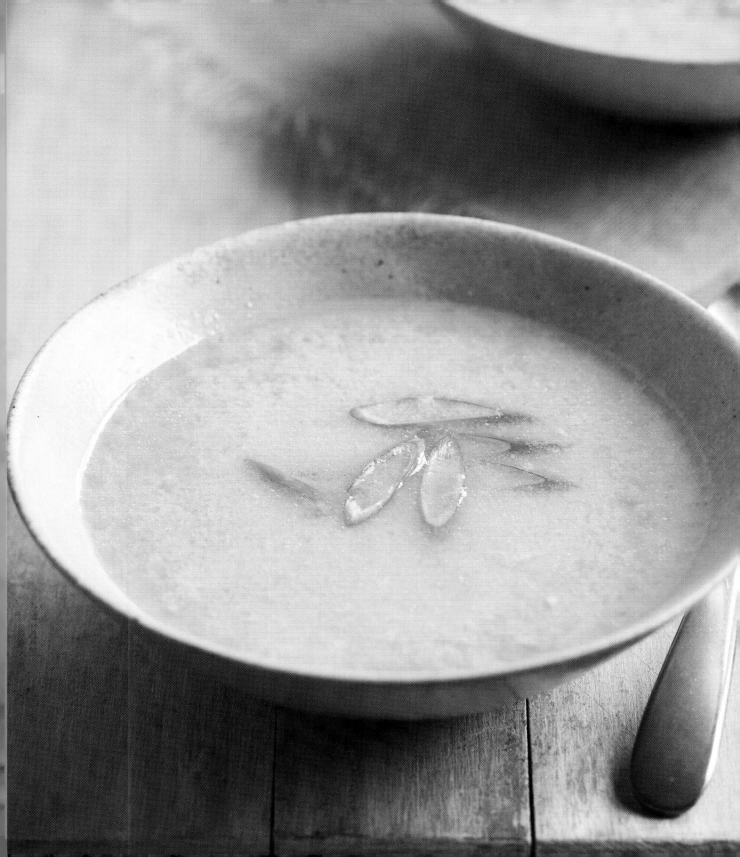

OYSTER STEW

NUT-FREE | EGG-FREE

PREP TIME: 5 minutes
COOK TIME: 8 minutes
TOTAL TIME: 13 minutes
SERVINGS: 3

Who says you need pricey fresh oysters to make an oyster stew that tastes as good as what you'd get at the best seafood restaurant? Ever the budget-minded chef, I just use canned oysters. This hearty soup is like seafood fast food!

¾ cup heavy cream

8 ounces canned oysters with their juice

4 tablespoons butter

1 tablespoon chopped fresh chives

1 tablespoon lemon juice

Salt and black pepper

Pour the heavy cream and the juice from the canned oysters in a 2-cup measuring container. Add water to make 2 cups liquid total. Set aside.

In a pot over medium heat, melt the butter. Add the chives, lemon juice, and the cream mixture. Bring to a boil over high heat. Reduce the heat to low and add the oysters. Cook until the oysters are heated through about 3 minutes, being careful not to overcook. Season with salt and black pepper to taste.

NOTES

Canned clams work well too if you prefer them to oysters.

NUTRITIONAL DATA

344 calories, 37g fat, 356mg sodium, 0g fiber, 2g carbohydrates, 1g protein

2g net carbs, 2% carbs, 1% protein, 97% fat

NO-BEAN CHILI

DAIRY-FREE | NUT-FREE | EGG-FREE | PALEO

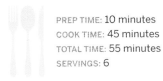

PREP TIME: 10 minutes
COOK TIME: 45 minutes
TOTAL TIME: 55 minutes
SERVINGS: 6

There's no need for beans in chili. They just add unnecessary carbs anyway. I like to ladle some of this meaty stew over spaghetti squash for a keto-friendly Cincinnati chili.

1 pound ground beef

2 (10-ounce) cans diced tomatoes with green chiles

2 tablespoons chili powder

1 teaspoon dried oregano

1 teaspoon onion powder

½ teaspoon salt

In a pot over medium-high heat, add the beef and cook, stirring and breaking up the meat with a wooden spoon, until browned, about 10 minutes. Add the canned tomatoes with chiles (including the liquid in the can) and 1¼ cups water, then stir in the chili powder, oregano, onion powder, and salt.

Reduce the heat, cover, and simmer for 35 to 40 minutes.

> **NUTRITIONAL DATA**
>
> 217 calories, 15g fat, 394mg sodium, 2g fiber, 5g carbohydrates, 14g protein
>
> 3g net carbs, 6% carbs, 28% protein, 66% fat

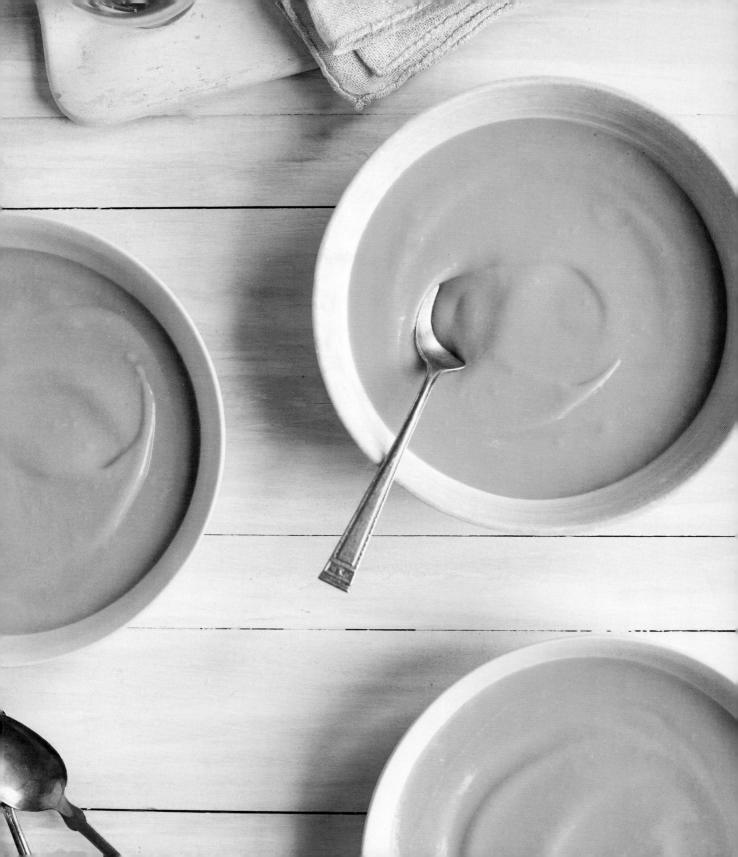

CREAMY AVOCADO SOUP

NUT-FREE | EGG-FREE

PREP TIME: 10 minutes
COOK TIME: 10 minutes
TOTAL TIME: 20 minutes
SERVINGS: 8

When it's too hot outside, chill out with this smart fat–filled, super-satiating soup. It's a great soup to take along for lunch as well, because it doesn't need to be heated.

3½ cups Slow-Cooked Roasted Bone Broth (page 26)

¼ cup lemon juice

1 teaspoon salt

4 large avocados, peeled and pitted

1½ cups heavy cream

Add the broth, lemon juice, and salt to a pot and bring to a boil over medium-high heat.

While the broth is heating, in a blender or food processor, puree the avocados with the cream until smooth.

Once the broth is boiling, remove from the heat and stir in the avocado mixture.

Refrigerate until chilled. Serve well chilled.

NOTES

An almond- or coconut-based coffee creamer can be used in place of the heavy cream for those avoiding dairy.

NUTRITIONAL DATA

321 calories, 31g fat, 677mg sodium, 6g fiber, 10g carbohydrates, 3g protein

4g net carbs, 5% carbs, 4% protein, 91% fat

CABBAGE AND GROUND BEEF SOUP

DAIRY-FREE | NUT-FREE | EGG-FREE PALEO. AIP

PREP TIME: 10 minutes
COOK TIME: 1 hour, 10 minutes
TOTAL TIME: 1 hour, 20 minutes
SERVINGS: 8

An ode to my Filipino roots, this recipe proves how versatile and satisfying cabbage is, especially with meat. You can even toss it together in the slow cooker after browning the meat.

1½ pounds ground beef

3 cloves garlic

1 large head cabbage, chopped

4 cups beef broth

1 tablespoon coconut aminos

1 teaspoon salt

Dash black pepper (omit for AIP)

In a large pot over medium heat, add the beef and garlic and cook, stirring and breaking up the meat with a wooden spoon, until browned, about 10 minutes.

Add the cabbage, 4 cups water, the broth, and the coconut aminos and season with the salt and pepper. Bring to a boil over high heat, then reduce the heat to medium-low, cover, and simmer for about 45 minutes.

NOTES

After browning the meat, it can be placed in a slow cooker with the rest of the ingredients and cooked on low for 6 to 8 hours or high for 3 to 4 hours.

NUTRITIONAL DATA

255 calories, 17g fat, 776mg sodium, 2g fiber, 7g carbohydrates, 17g protein

8g net carbs, 8% carbs, 28% protein, 64% fat

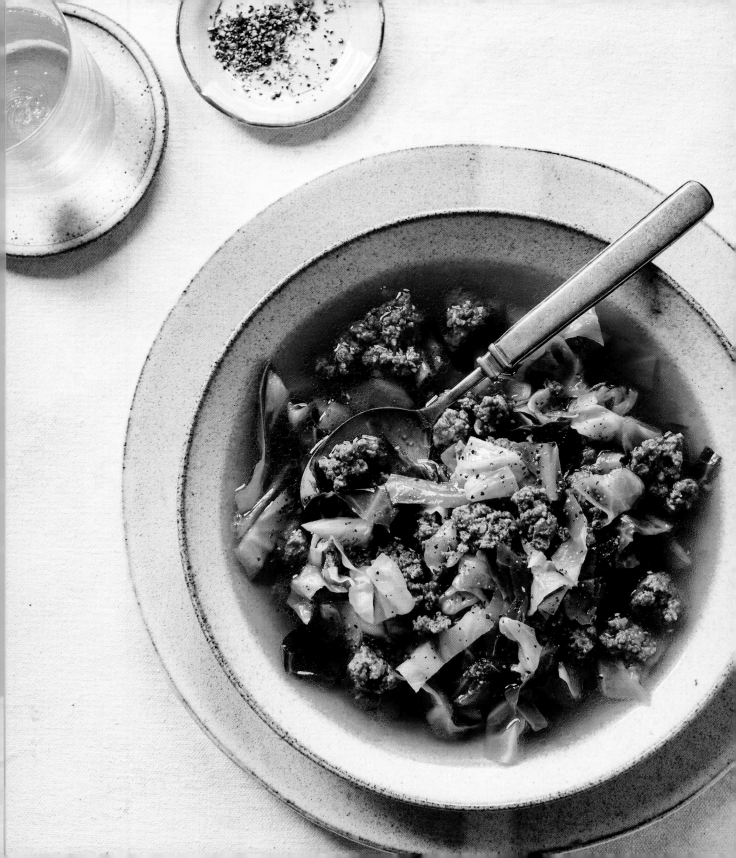

CREAM OF MUSHROOM SOUP

NUT-FREE | EGG-FREE

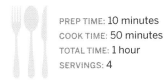

PREP TIME: 10 minutes
COOK TIME: 50 minutes
TOTAL TIME: 1 hour
SERVINGS: 4

Somehow this version of the classic soup manages to be more satisfying, even though the mouthfeel is thinner because there's no high-carb thickener. It feels more like a soup and less like a gravy!

2 tablespoons extra-virgin olive oil or butter

8 ounces white or baby bella mushrooms, sliced

2 stalks celery, diced

2 cups Slow-Cooked Roasted Bone Broth (page 26)

1½ cups heavy cream

Salt and black pepper

Heat the oil in a pan over medium heat. Add the mushrooms and celery and cook, stirring, until the celery is tender, 12 to 15 minutes. Add the broth, bring to a simmer, and cook for about 15 minutes.

Stir in the cream, then bring to a boil. Reduce the heat to maintain a simmer and cook, stirring occasionally, for 10 minutes more. Season to taste with salt and black pepper.

NOTES

Two to 4 tablespoons chopped onion can be cooked with the celery and mushrooms.

NUTRITIONAL DATA

388 calories, 40g fat, 468mg sodium, 0g fiber, 4g carbohydrates, 4g protein

4g net carbs, 4% carbs, 4% protein, 92% fat

PUMPKIN SOUP

DAIRY-FREE | NUT-FREE | EGG-FREE | PALEO, AIP

PREP TIME: 5 minutes
COOK TIME: 15 minutes
TOTAL TIME: 20 minutes
SERVINGS: 6

Don't let pumpkin spice lattes hog the spotlight. Pumpkin soup should be enjoyed year-round. Pumpkin is the only vegetable I buy canned because it's easier that way and still super-rich in vitamin A.

15 ounces canned pumpkin puree

1¾ cups coconut milk (one 14-ounce can)

1¾ cups Slow-Cooked Roasted Bone Broth (page 26)

6 slices bacon, cooked and chopped

1 teaspoon dried sage

½ teaspoon salt

Black pepper (omit for AIP)

Whisk together the pumpkin puree, coconut milk, and broth in a medium pot. Stir in the bacon and sage. Cook over medium heat for 12 to 15 minutes. Season with the salt and black pepper to taste.

NOTES

Almond milk or a mix of heavy cream and water can be used in place of the coconut milk.

NUTRITIONAL DATA

249 calories, 23g fat, 591mg sodium, 2g fiber, 8g carbohydrates, 5g protein

6g net carbs, 10% carbs, 8% protein, 82% fat

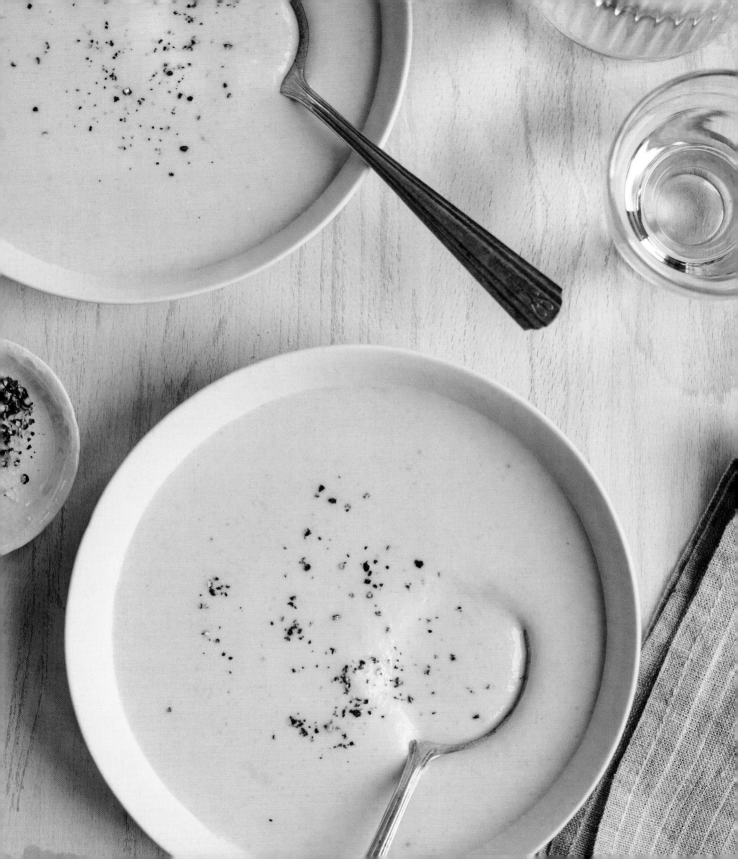

YELLOW SQUASH SOUP

PREP TIME: 10 minutes
COOK TIME: 15 minutes
TOTAL TIME: 25 minutes
SERVINGS: 4

NUT-FREE | EGG-FREE

Cream cheese and squash? Hey, if cream cheese works well with sushi, wait until you give this simple soup a taste. Pair it with a tossed salad for a light lunch.

1 pound yellow squash, thinly sliced

1¾ cup Slow-Cooked Roasted Bone Broth (page 26)

¼ cup coconut oil

4 ounces cream cheese, softened

¼ teaspoon dried thyme

Salt and black pepper

Add the squash, broth, and coconut oil to a medium pot. Bring to a boil over medium-high heat. Reduce the heat to maintain a simmer, cover, and cook until the squash is tender, about 10 minutes. Remove from the heat and add the cream cheese. Allow to cool slightly.

Using an immersion blender, blend the mixture until smooth (or let cool and blend in a regular blender in batches). Stir in salt and black pepper to taste.

NOTES

About ¼ cup chopped onion can be added with the squash for added flavor, and will only increase the carbs in each serving by about 1 gram.

NUTRITIONAL DATA

173 calories, 14g fat, 564mg sodium, 1g fiber, 6g carbohydrates, 6g protein

5g net carbs, 12% carbs, 14% protein, 74% fat

ROASTED BRUSSELS WITH BACON SOUP

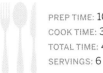

PREP TIME: 10 minutes
COOK TIME: 30 minutes
TOTAL TIME: 40 minutes
SERVINGS: 6

DAIRY-FREE | NUT-FREE | EGG-FREE | PALEO, AIP

I just love Brussels sprouts, especially when they are paired with pieces of bacon. Roasting them with a drizzling of olive oil adds a touch of sweetness to them and a richer flavor.

1 pound Brussels sprouts, halved lengthwise

2 tablespoons extra-virgin olive oil

6 slices bacon

½ cup chopped onion

4 cups Slow-Cooked Roasted Bone Broth (page 26)

½ teaspoon salt

Preheat the oven to 425°F.

Place the Brussels sprouts cut side down on a rimmed baking sheet and drizzle with the oil. Bake for 25 minutes, flipping after about 12 minutes.

While the Brussels are baking, cook the bacon in large pot. When completely cooked, remove the bacon from the pot with a slotted spoon and set on paper towels to drain.

In the same pot, add the onion and cook in the bacon grease, stirring, until translucent, about 5 minutes. Stir in the broth and salt, bring to a boil, then reduce the heat and simmer for about 5 minutes.

Chop the cooked bacon and add half to the soup, along with the roasted Brussels sprouts. Allow the soup to simmer for another 5 minutes.

Using an immersion blender, blend the soup until smooth (or let cool and then blend in a traditional blender). Serve with the remaining bacon pieces sprinkled on top.

NOTES

Parchment paper or a silicone baking mat can be used for easier cleanup when roasting the Brussels sprouts.

NUTRITIONAL DATA

178 calories, 13g fat, 932mg sodium, 3g fiber, 8g carbohydrates, 6g protein

5g net carbs, 12% carbs, 15% protein, 73% fat

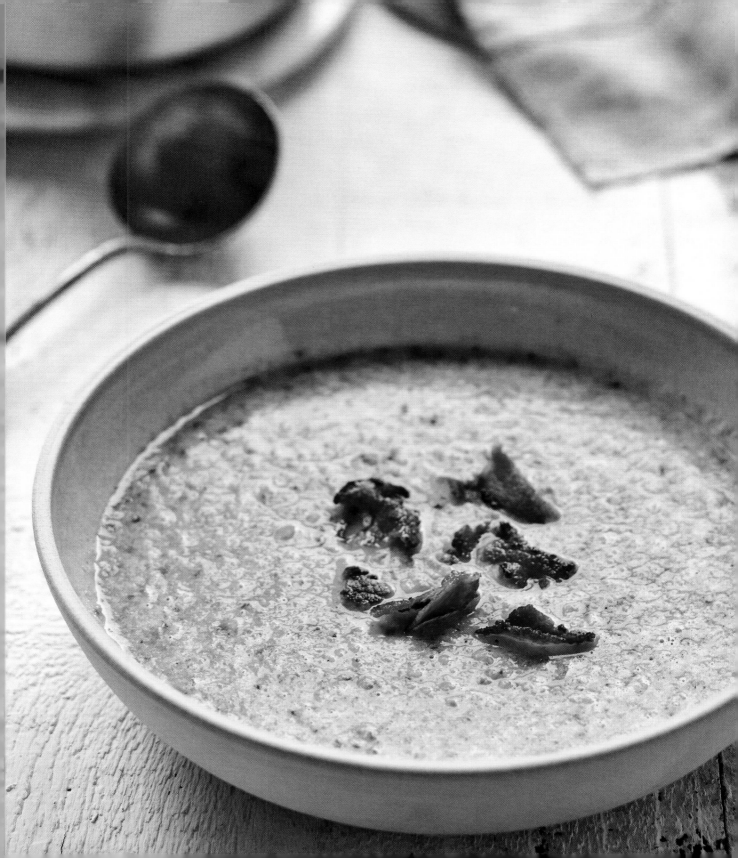

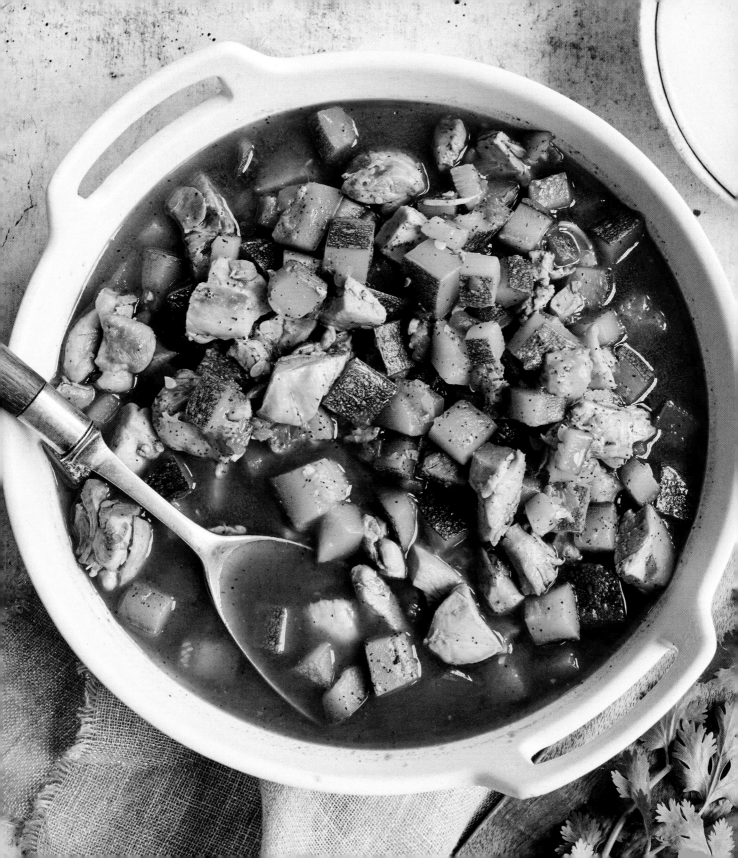

CHICKEN CHILI

DAIRY-FREE | NUT-FREE | EGG-FREE | PALEO

PREP TIME: 10 minutes
COOK TIME: 20 minutes
TOTAL TIME: 30 minutes
SERVINGS: 6

You know zucchini are a great replacement for noodles, fries, and chips. But did you know they're an excellent substitute for beans too? Just dice them so they are a similar size! This keto chili is a great way to repurpose leftover chicken.

2 cups Slow-Cooked Roasted Bone Broth (page 26)

2 medium zucchini, diced

1 (4-ounce) can chopped green chiles, or 3 fresh chiles, chopped

1 tablespoon chili powder

2 cups diced cooked chicken thigh meat

Salt

Fresh cilantro (optional), for garnish

In a large pot, combine the broth, zucchini, green chiles (including the liquid in the can), and chili powder and bring to a boil over high heat. Reduce the heat to maintain a simmer and cook, stirring occasionally, to allow the flavors to blend, about 5 minutes.

Stir in the chicken and heat throughout, about 5 minutes. Season to taste with salt. If desired, sprinkle with cilantro.

NOTES

Coconut oil can be added to each serving to increase the fat content.

Great add-ins are diced bell peppers, diced tomatoes, and cumin.

If you use fresh chiles, they can be roasted first for better flavor.

Freezer option: Freeze cooled chili in freezer containers. To use, partially thaw in the refrigerator overnight. Reheat in a saucepan, stirring occasionally and adding a little water if needed.

NUTRITIONAL DATA

243 calories, 8g fat, 675mg sodium, 1g fiber, 3g carbohydrates, 37g protein

2g net carbs, 4% carbs, 65% protein, 32% fat

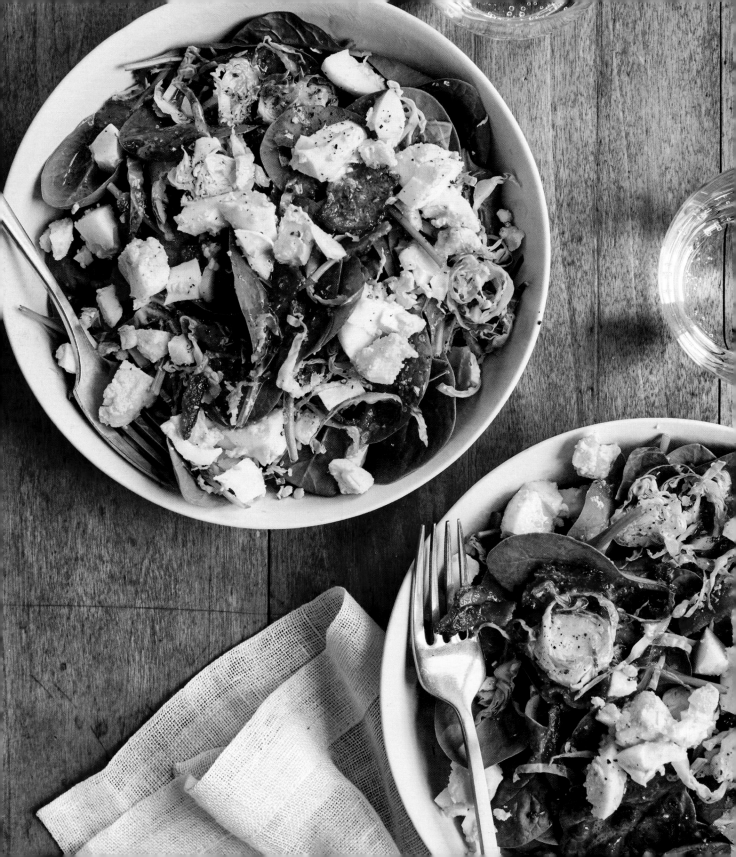

SALADS

Baby Vegetable Mixed Salad 50
Creamy Dill-Cucumber Salad 52
Broccoli Salad 53
Summer Squash Salad 53
Radish Salad 56
Sour Cream–Lettuce Salad 57
Wedge Salad 58
Baby Kale Salad 58
Spinach-Bacon Salad 61
Green Bean–Tomato Salad 62
Salmon-Cucumber Salad 64
Cabbage Salad 65
Pesto Chicken Salad 67

BABY VEGETABLE MIXED SALAD

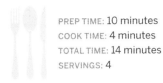

PREP TIME: 10 minutes
COOK TIME: 4 minutes
TOTAL TIME: 14 minutes
SERVINGS: 4

DAIRY-FREE | NUT-FREE | EGG-FREE | PALEO, AIP IF MODIFIED

A mix of tender young vegetables are blended together with a simple red wine vinaigrette dressing. Add some grilled chicken or steak to make it a meal.

1 medium yellow squash, sliced and quartered (about 2 cups)

1 cup sliced young green beans, cut into bite-size pieces (use zucchini if AIP)

7½ cups (5 ounces) baby spinach

¼ cup extra-virgin olive oil

2 tablespoons red wine vinegar

Salt and black pepper (omit pepper for AIP)

Steam the squash and green beans until crisp-tender, 3 to 4 minutes.

Place the steamed vegetables in a large bowl and add the spinach. Stir to combine.

In a small bowl, whisk together the oil and vinegar. Add salt and black pepper to taste. Pour over the vegetables and mix well.

NOTES

The green beans can be replaced with zucchini or radishes if desired.

NUTRITIONAL DATA

145 calories, 13g fat, 104mg sodium, 2g fiber, 4g carbohydrates, 2g protein

2g net carbs, 6% carbs, 6% protein, 88% fat

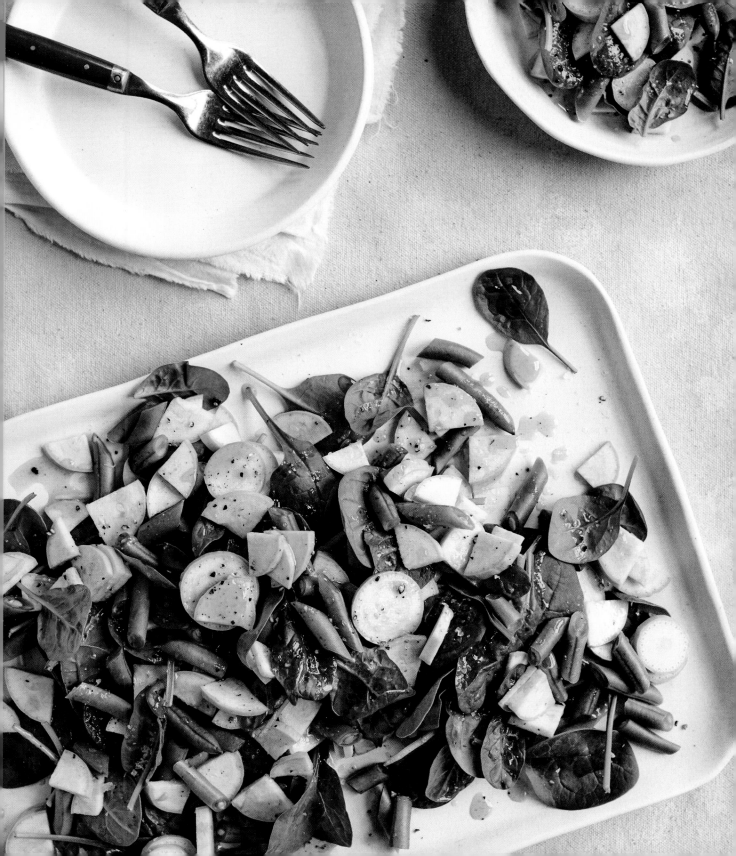

CREAMY DILL-CUCUMBER SALAD

NUT-FREE | EGG-FREE

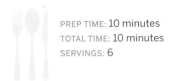

PREP TIME: 10 minutes
TOTAL TIME: 10 minutes
SERVINGS: 6

Usually, cucumbers take a back seat to other salad mainstays, but in this salad, they shine. The creamy dill dressing has the perfect touch of sweetness. Bring it along for a picnic or summer potluck.

3 medium cucumbers, sliced

¼ cup chopped fresh dill

1 cup sour cream

¼ cup apple cider vinegar

12 drops liquid stevia extract

½ teaspoon salt

Dash black pepper

Combine the cucumbers and dill in a large bowl.

In a separate bowl, whisk together the sour cream, vinegar, stevia, salt, and black pepper until well combined. Stir the sour cream mixture into the cucumber and dill.

Chill for at least 2 hours before serving.

NOTES

Chopped red onion can be added.

NUTRITIONAL DATA

146 calories, 11g fat, 343mg sodium, 1g fiber, 6g carbohydrates, 2g protein

5g net carbs, 16% carbs, 6% protein, 78% fat

BROCCOLI SALAD

DAIRY-FREE | NUT-FREE | PALEO

PREP TIME: 10 minutes	COOK TIME: 20 minutes
TOTAL TIME: 30 minutes	SERVINGS: 8

You have to love raw broccoli if you're going to enjoy this simple salad, but the tangy dressing soaks into the florets. Share it with friends and family at summer gatherings.

½ cup mayonnaise

1 tablespoon apple cider vinegar

15 drops liquid stevia extract (or to taste)

20 ounces broccoli, cut into florets

8 ounces bacon, chopped and cooked until crisp

In a large bowl, combine the mayonnaise, vinegar, and stevia. Toss in the broccoli and bacon until well coated with the dressing.

NOTES

Grated cheddar cheese works well with about ½ cup mixed in. Sunflower seeds also make a nice topping.

NUTRITIONAL DATA

237 calories, 21g fat, 300mg sodium, 1g fiber, 5g carbohydrates, 5g protein

4g net carbs, 7% carbs, 9% protein, 84% fat

SUMMER SQUASH SALAD

DAIRY-FREE | NUT-FREE | EGG-FREE | PALEO

PREP TIME: 10 minutes	COOK TIME: 8 minutes
TOTAL TIME: 18 minutes	SERVINGS: 4

There's a good chance someone will be bringing coleslaw to the barbecue, so change things up with this easy salad. If you have a garden, these two squashes will be prime for picking in summer.

1 large summer squash

1 large zucchini

½ cup cherry or grape tomatoes

1 batch Italian Dressing (page 86)

Slice the squash and zucchini in half lengthwise and then in slices. Place in a steamer over boiling water. Cover and steam for 2 to 3 minutes, then place in cold water to stop the cooking. Drain well and place in a medium bowl.

Cut the tomatoes in half. Add to the squash and zucchini along with the dressing. Toss to coat. This can be served chilled or at room temperature.

NUTRITIONAL DATA

116 calories, 10g fat, 8mg sodium, 1g fiber, 4g carbohydrates, 1g protein

3g net carbs, 11% carbs, 4% protein, 85% fat

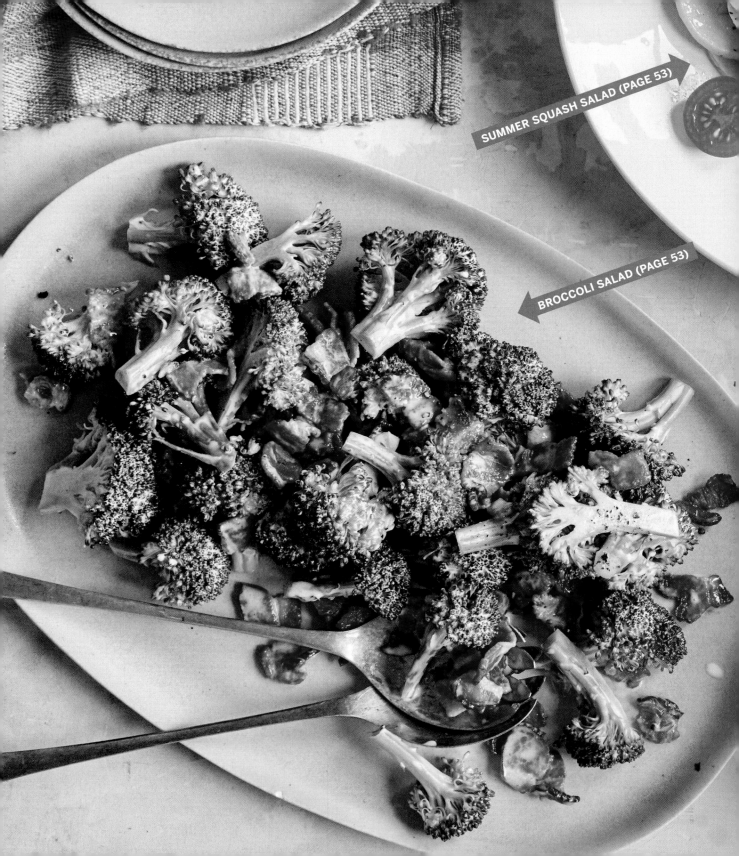

SUMMER SQUASH SALAD (PAGE 53)

BROCCOLI SALAD (PAGE 53)

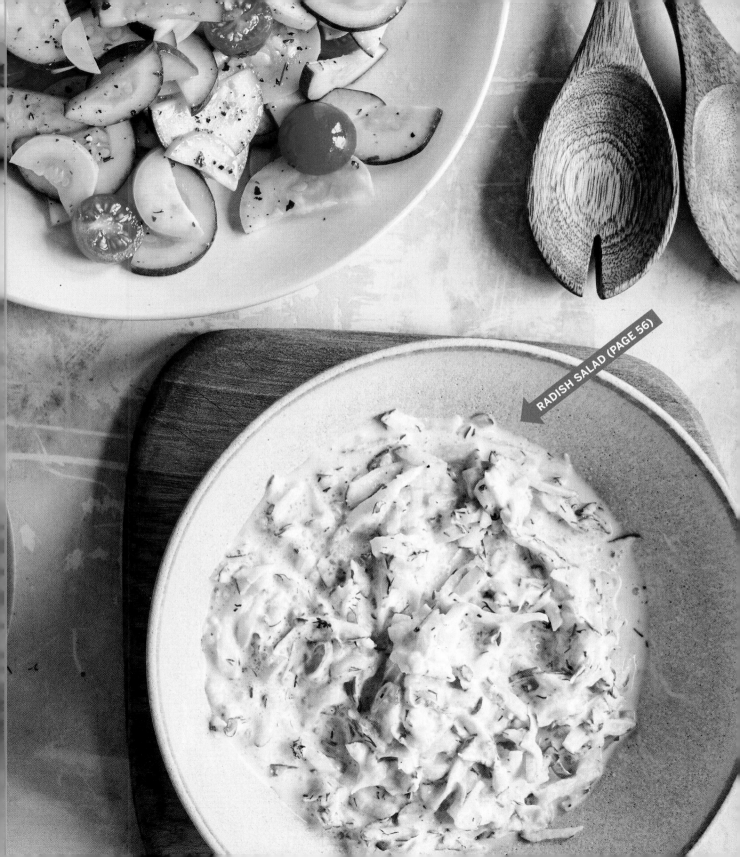

RADISH SALAD (PAGE 56)

RADISH SALAD

NUT-FREE | EGG-FREE

PREP TIME: 20 minutes
TOTAL TIME: 20 minutes
SERVINGS: 8

Old World tradition meets New World sensibilities, without sacrificing taste. It's a perfect pairing of cream and crunch, filling yet light, and is ideal for summer barbecues. Try serving it on a bed of lettuce.

16 ounces cottage cheese

12 ounces radishes, grated

2 green onions, thinly sliced

½ cup sour cream

1 teaspoon chopped fresh dill

½ teaspoon salt

Black pepper (optional)

Place the cottage cheese in a fine mesh strainer over a bowl and let sit for about 15 minutes to remove any excess liquid.

In a new bowl, mix the cottage cheese with the radishes, onions, sour cream, dill, salt, and pepper (if desired), and chill for at least 30 minutes.

NOTES

Add chopped green or red peppers, cucumber, or celery to the salad.

If desired, the radishes can be sliced instead of grated.

NUTRITIONAL DATA

91 calories, 5g fat, 380mg sodium, 1g fiber, 4g carbohydrates, 7g protein

1g net carbs, 14% carbs, 33% protein, 53% fat

SOUR CREAM–LETTUCE SALAD

NUT-FREE

PREP TIME: 15 minutes
TOTAL TIME: 15 minutes
SERVINGS: 4

Warm up your taste buds with this simple salad drenched in a tangy cream dressing. It's just enough to satisfy without taking too much away from the main entrée.

1 head iceberg lettuce

½ medium lemon

½ cup sour cream

2 teaspoons chopped fresh parsley

½ teaspoon salt

Black pepper (optional)

2 hard-cooked large eggs

Liquid stevia extract (optional)

Tear the lettuce into bite-size pieces and place in a medium bowl.

Grate the zest of the lemon and then squeeze the juice. In a small bowl, combine the sour cream, parsley, salt, and pepper (if desired), lemon zest, and lemon juice. If needed, add a touch of sweetener. Pour the dressing over the lettuce in the bowl.

Cut the hard-cooked eggs in half and remove the yolks. Finely dice the whites and sprinkle over the sour cream dressing.

Push the yolks through a fine-mesh strainer over the bowl and sprinkle over the top of the salad. Alternatively, the yolks can be finely chopped with a knife and sprinkled on.

NOTES

Sliced cucumbers, celery, radishes, or peppers can be added to the salad.

NUTRITIONAL DATA

109 calories, 7g fat, 358mg sodium, 1g fiber, 6g carbohydrates, 4g protein

5g net carbs, 20% carbs, 16% protein, 64% fat

WEDGE SALAD

NUT-FREE | EGG-FREE

> **PREP TIME:** 10 minutes　　**Total Time:** 10 minutes
> **SERVINGS:** 4

While iceberg lettuce isn't the most nutrient-dense veggie on the planet, sometimes you just crave something you grew up eating for years at restaurants and your friends' houses. So, keep it simple with a classic wedge salad.

1 head iceberg lettuce
½ batch Blue Cheese Dressing (page 94)
1 tomato, diced
4 slices bacon, cooked until crisp and chopped
1 cup blue cheese crumbles

Cut the lettuce into 4 wedges. Place each wedge on a plate. Drizzle the blue cheese dressing over each wedge. Sprinkle the tomato, bacon, and blue cheese crumbles on top.

NOTES

To make it eat more like a meal, sprinkle a chopped hard-cooked egg onto each serving.

NUTRITIONAL DATA

313 calories, 25g fat, 957mg sodium, 1g fiber, 7g carbohydrates, 15g protein
6g net carbs, 8% carbs, 19% protein, 73% fat

BABY KALE SALAD

DAIRY-FREE | EGG-FREE | PALEO

> **PREP TIME:** 10 minutes　　**COOK TIME:** 5 minutes
> **TOTAL TIME:** 15 minutes　　**SERVINGS:** 6

Full of healthy fats and nutrient-rich kale, this salad proves that mega-healthy and an abundance of flavor can coexist.

5 ounces baby kale (about 1 packed cup)
8 slices bacon, cooked and chopped
½ cup sliced almonds
1 medium avocado, diced
½ batch Balsamic Vinaigrette (page 93)

In a large bowl, combine the baby kale, bacon, almonds, and avocado. Stir in the vinaigrette.

NOTES

Top each serving with grated Parmesan cheese if desired.

NUTRITIONAL DATA

405 calories, 39g fat, 512mg sodium, 3g fiber, 8g carbohydrates,7g protein
5g net carbs, 5% carbs, 7% protein, 88% fat

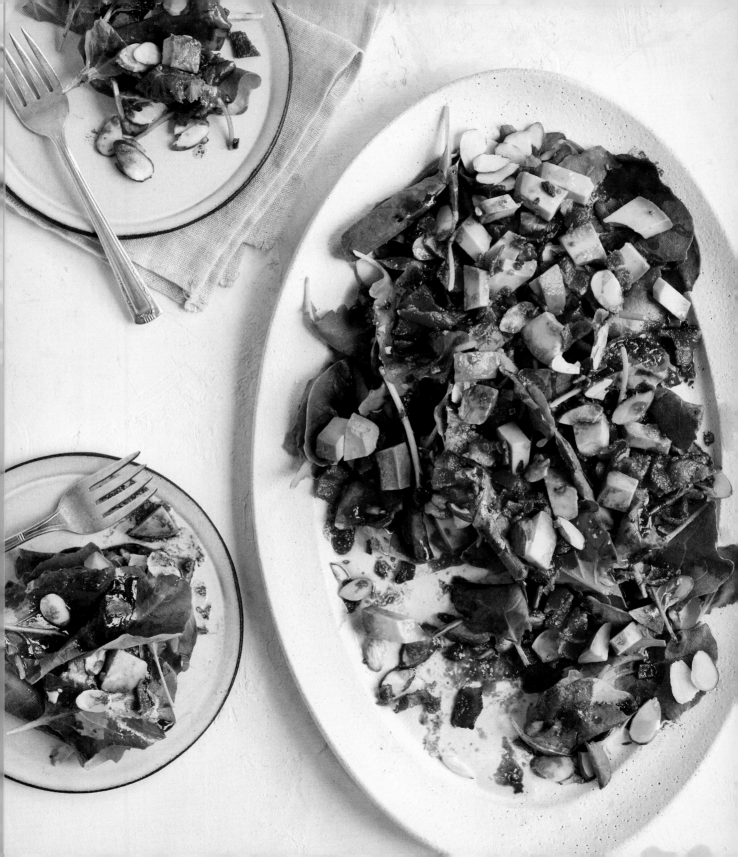

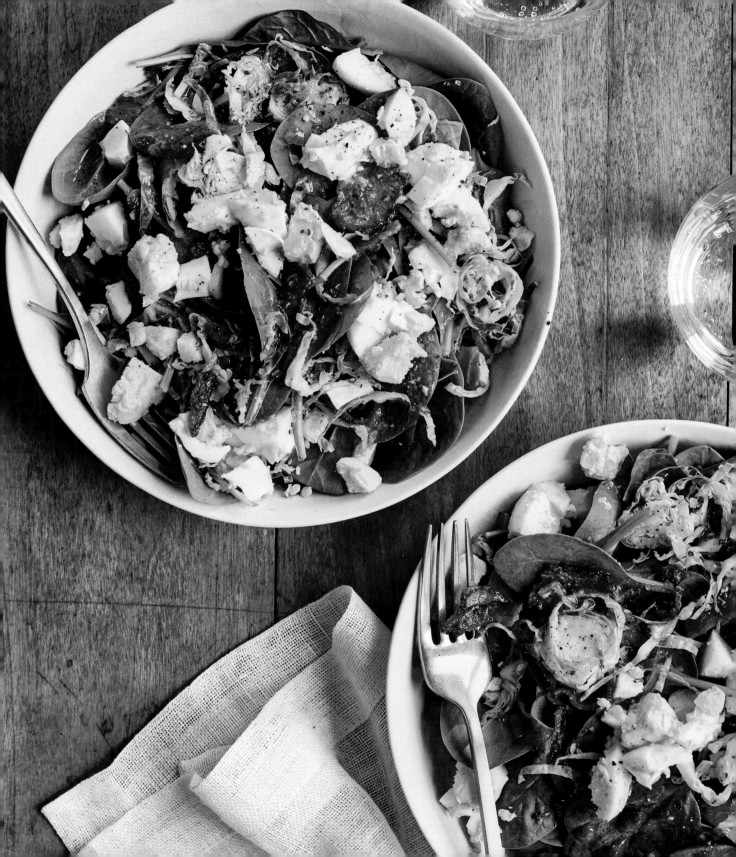

SPINACH-BACON SALAD

DAIRY-FREE | NUT-FREE | PALEO

PREP TIME: 10 minutes
COOK TIME: 5 minutes
TOTAL TIME: 20 minutes
SERVINGS: 2

This warm spinach salad features a high-fat dressing made with bacon fat and vinegar. Add cooked chicken or steak for a complete meal.

7½ cups (5 ounces) baby spinach

2 ounces bacon, chopped

2 hard-boiled eggs, chopped

¼ cup apple cider vinegar

2 teaspoons Dijon mustard

Salt and black pepper

Place the spinach in a medium salad bowl. Set aside.

Cook the bacon in a skillet over medium heat, stirring occasionally, until crispy, about 5 minutes. Remove from the pan and place on paper towels to cool.

Remove the pan with the bacon grease from the heat. Stir in the vinegar and mustard and season with salt and black pepper to taste. Pour over the baby spinach and toss to coat. Top with the reserved chopped bacon and eggs.

NOTES

Sliced mushrooms or shredded Brussels sprouts can be added.

NUTRITIONAL DATA

221 calories, 17g fat, 363mg sodium, 1g fiber, 4g carbohydrates, 12g protein

3g net carbs, 6% carbs, 23% protein, 72% fat

GREEN BEAN–TOMATO SALAD

PREP TIME: 10 minutes
COOK TIME: 10 minutes
TOTAL TIME: 20 minutes
SERVINGS: 6

DAIRY-FREE | NUT-FREE | EGG-FREE | PALEO

The green of the string beans with the red of the cherry tomatoes and purple hue on the onion make this a colorful dish. But it's kept simple by topping with a basic Italian dressing.

1 pound green beans, cut into slices
½ cup grape tomatoes, quartered
½ red onion, chopped
½ cup Italian Dressing (page 86)

Place the green beans in a medium saucepan and cover with water. Bring to a boil, then cook until crisp-tender, 2 to 4 minutes. Drain the green beans and rinse with cool water to stop the cooking. Transfer to large bowl.

Add the tomatoes, red onion, and dressing. Toss to coat.

NOTES

Black olives make a great add-in.

Tender young green beans work best in a salad.

NUTRITIONAL DATA
94 calories, 7g fat, 103mg sodium, 2 fiber, 6g carbohydrates, 1g protein
4g net carbs, 19% carbs, 5% protein, 76% fat

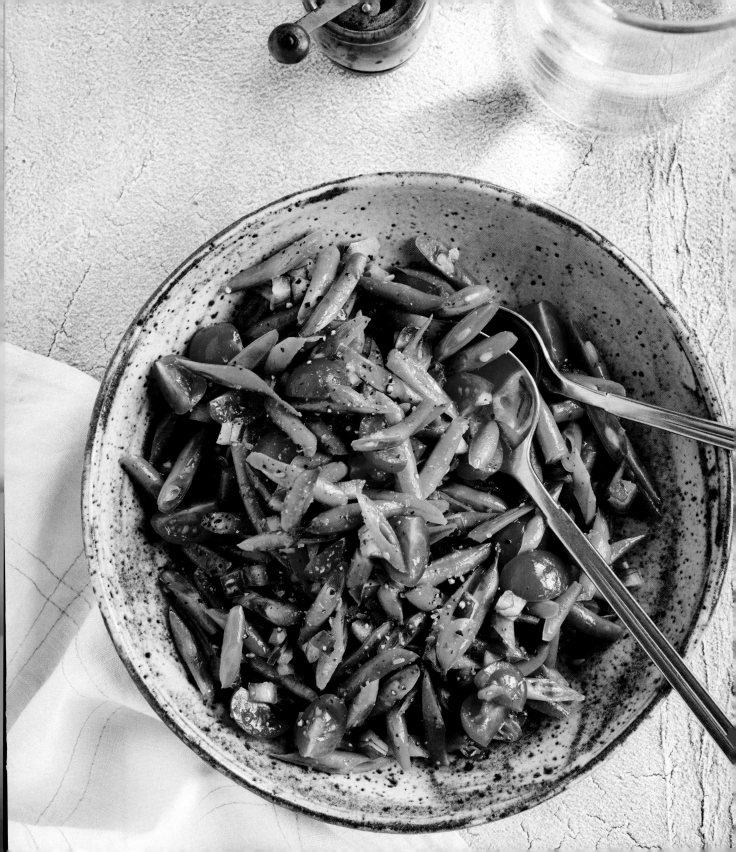

SALMON-CUCUMBER SALAD

PREP TIME: 5 minutes
TOTAL TIME: 5 minutes
SERVINGS: 6

DAIRY-FREE | NUT-FREE | PALEO

Love tuna fish but concerned about mercury, or just want to change it up? Try canned wild salmon. It can be served in lettuce wraps, or it goes great with chopped cucumbers. A crunchy healthy dose of omega-3s made delectable thanks to the homemade dill seasoning.

2 (5-ounce) cans wild salmon

1 English cucumber, peeled and seeded

¼ cup mayonnaise, plus more if needed

1 teaspoon dried dill (or 1 tablespoon fresh)

½ teaspoon onion powder

Drain the liquid from the salmon, then place it in a medium bowl. Break the fish into small pieces with a fork. Chop the cucumber into small pieces and stir into the salmon.

Stir in the mayonnaise, dill, and onion powder, adding more mayonnaise if desired.

NOTES

Celery can be used instead of cucumber. A touch of lemon juice is also a nice addition.

NUTRITIONAL DATA

137 calories, 9g fat, 240mg sodium, 0g fiber, 2g carbohydrates, 11g protein

2g net carbs, 6% carbs, 33% protein, 61% fat

CABBAGE SALAD

DAIRY-FREE | NUT-FREE | PALEO

PREP TIME: 10 minutes
TOTAL TIME: 10 minutes
SERVINGS: 8

Cabbage is a superfood that's high in immune-boosting vitamin C. Making a coleslaw without carrots makes it more keto-friendly. Serve it as a side with burgers or use it to top barbecued shredded pork or chicken.

1 head cabbage, shredded or grated

¼ cup apple cider vinegar

¼ cup mayonnaise

½ teaspoon celery seed

**¼ teaspoon liquid stevia extract or
2 tablespoons granular sweetener**

Salt and black pepper

Place the cabbage in a large bowl.

In a separate bowl, mix the vinegar, mayonnaise, celery seed, stevia, and salt and black pepper to taste. Pour over the cabbage and toss to coat.

Chill for at least 2 hours before serving.

NOTES

A couple tablespoons of chopped onion can be added.

NUTRITIONAL DATA

78 calories, 5g fat, 138mg sodium, 2g fiber,
6g carbohydrates, 1g protein

4g net carbs, 7% carbs, 2% protein, 92% fat

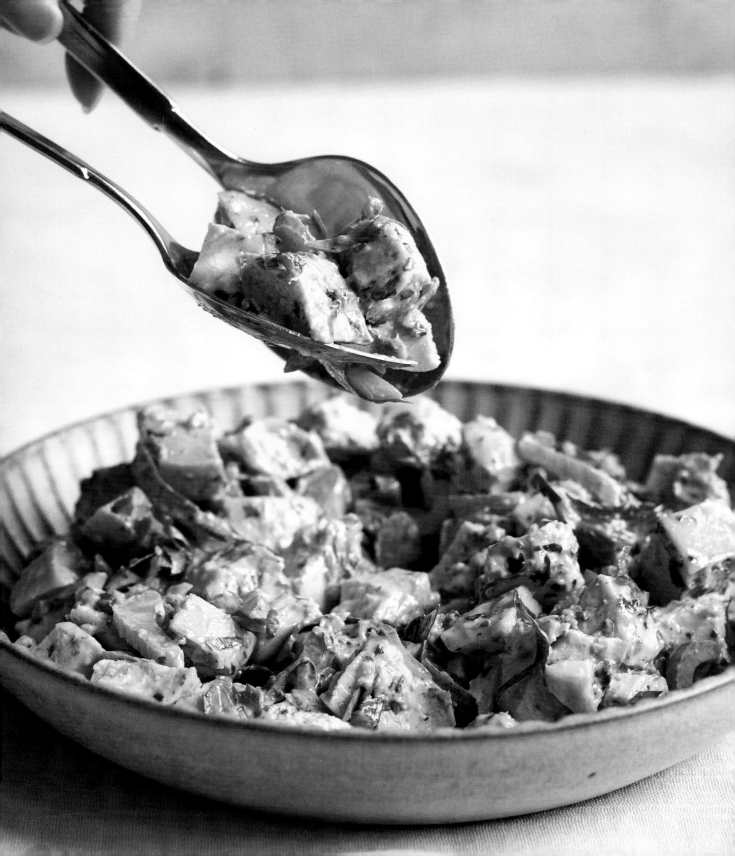

PESTO CHICKEN SALAD

DAIRY-FREE | NUT-FREE | PALEO

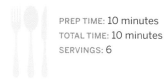

PREP TIME: 10 minutes
TOTAL TIME: 10 minutes
SERVINGS: 6

An Italian spin on Thai-style lettuce or cabbage wraps. The pesto is easy to make but not overpowering. Make enough of these, and you won't need an entrée to go with it.

2 cups cubed cooked chicken

Basil Pesto (page 92)

½ cup mayonnaise

⅓ cup chopped celery (about 2 stalks)

Salt and black pepper

In a large bowl, combine the chicken, pesto, mayonnaise, celery, and salt and black pepper to taste. Stir until well combined.

NOTES

This works well in a lettuce or cabbage wrap.

NUTRITIONAL DATA

405 calories, 36g fat, 448mg sodium, 1g fiber, 3g carbohydrates, 16g protein

2g net carbs, 2% carbs, 16% protein, 82% fat

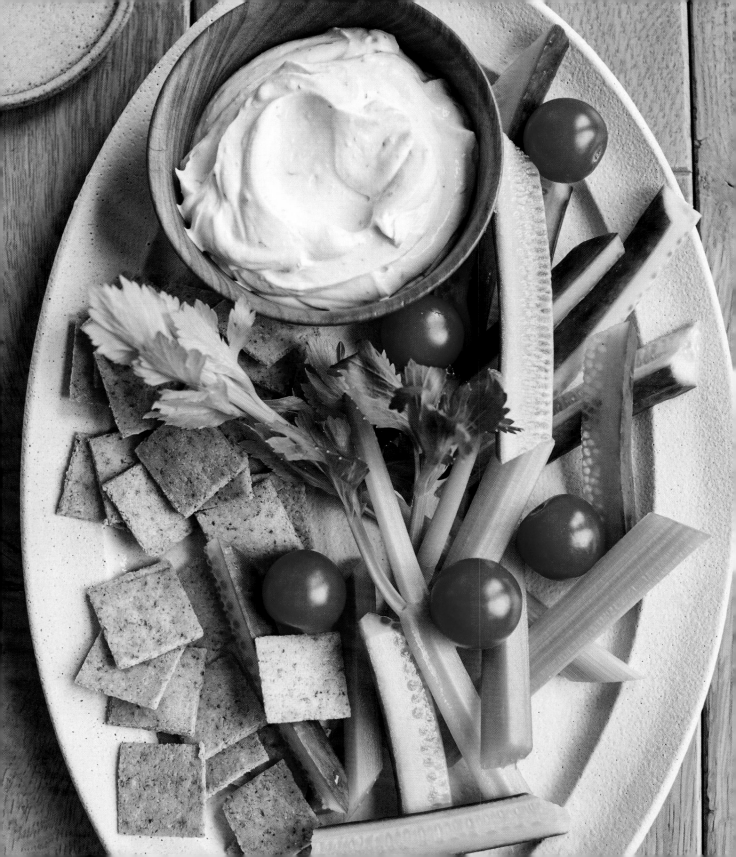

APPETIZERS AND SNACKS

Almond Flour Bread 70

Almond Cheese 72

Mexican Cheese Dip 73

Nutty Crackers 76

Stuffed Cucumber Slices 77

Cheese Ball 78

Avocado Deviled Eggs 79

Seasoned Tortilla Chips 80

Sour Cream and Onion Dip 83

ALMOND FLOUR BREAD

PREP TIME: 10 minutes
COOK TIME: 45 minutes
TOTAL TIME: 55 minutes
SERVINGS: 16

DAIRY-FREE | PALEO

A guilt-free bread that's a meal in itself. Bread has never been so satisfying and healthy: ultra-low-carb with moderate protein and ample healthy fats. Have two slices without the worry of insulin spikes!

2 cups blanched almond flour

1 teaspoon baking soda

¼ teaspoon salt

¼ cup coconut oil, melted if needed to liquefy

4 large eggs, at room temperature

1 teaspoon apple cider vinegar

Preheat the oven to 325°F. Grease an 8 × 4-inch loaf pan or line with parchment paper.

Combine the almond flour, baking soda, and salt in medium bowl. Set aside.

In a large bowl, whisk together the coconut oil, eggs, and vinegar. Add the almond flour mixture and stir until just combined. Spread into the prepared loaf pan.

Bake for 40 to 45 minutes, until the bread is golden and a toothpick or knife inserted into the center comes out clean.

NOTES

For best results, the batter should be baked as soon as possible once the dry ingredients are combined with the wet ingredients, so be sure to have the oven preheated by that time.

Herbs, spices, and seeds can be included to add flavor and create different varieties.

NUTRITIONAL DATA

129 calories, 12g fat, 125mg sodium, 1g fiber, 3g carbohydrates, 5g protein

2g net carbs, 6% carbs, 15% protein, 79% fat

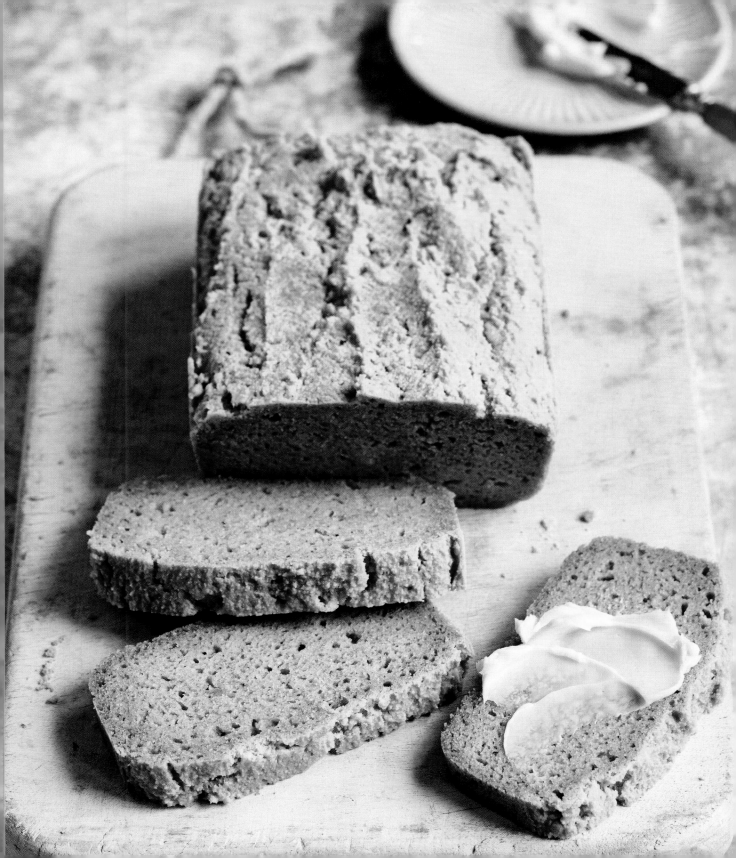

ALMOND CHEESE

DAIRY-FREE | EGG-FREE | PALEO

PREP TIME: 15 minutes
COOK TIME: 35 minutes
SOAK/DRAIN TIME: 16 hours
TOTAL TIME: 16 hours 50 minutes
SERVINGS: 8

It may feel like you're creating real cheese when straining the mix with a cheesecloth. But this is a fantastic alternative to the real thing if you want to eliminate dairy, and it's easy to make at home.

1 cup blanched almonds (about 4½ ounces)
2½ tablespoons lemon juice
2½ tablespoons extra-virgin olive oil
½ teaspoon garlic powder
1 teaspoon sea salt

Soak the almonds in water for at least 8 hours.

Drain the almonds. Place the nuts in a food processor or blender with the lemon juice, oil, garlic powder, and salt. Puree until the mixture is smooth, adding small amounts of water as needed.

Line a fine-mesh strainer with cheesecloth and place over a bowl. Transfer the almond mixture into the cheesecloth. Allow the mixture to drain in the refrigerator for at least 8 hours.

Preheat the oven to 350°F. Lightly grease a sheet pan or line it with parchment paper.

Shape the drained almond mixture into a cheese shape such as a ball or log on the prepared sheet pan. Bake for about 35 minutes, or until set to desired doneness.

Allow to cool, then store, covered, in the refrigerator. Serve chilled.

NOTES

Herbs and spices can be added to change up the taste. The shaped almond mixture can also be coated with chopped nuts before baking.

Small bits of the almond cheese are perfect for adding cheesy flavor to a tossed salad or a quiche for those avoiding dairy.

NUTRITIONAL DATA

133 calories, 13g fat, 295mg sodium, 2g fiber, 3g carbohydrates, 3g protein

2g net carbs, 3% carbs, 9% protein, 88% fat

MEXICAN CHEESE DIP

PREP TIME: 5 minutes
COOK TIME: 10 minutes
TOTAL TIME: 15 minutes
SERVINGS: 6

NUT-FREE | EGG-FREE

Sauce or dip: you choose! When the family complains yet again about eating plain steamed veggies, this is the perfect thing to drown them in.

¾ cup heavy cream

4 ounces sharp cheddar cheese, finely shredded

4 ounces canned chopped green chiles, undrained

¼ teaspoon ground cumin

¼ teaspoon onion powder

¼ teaspoon salt

In a saucepan over low heat, combine the heavy cream, cheese, chiles, cumin, onion powder, and salt and cook, stirring often, until the cheese is melted. Serve warm.

NOTES

Water can be added to thin out the dip if needed.

NUTRITIONAL DATA

138 calories, 12g fat, 216mg sodium, 0g fiber, 1g carbohydrates, 4g protein

1g net carbs, 3% carbs, 13% protein, 84% fat

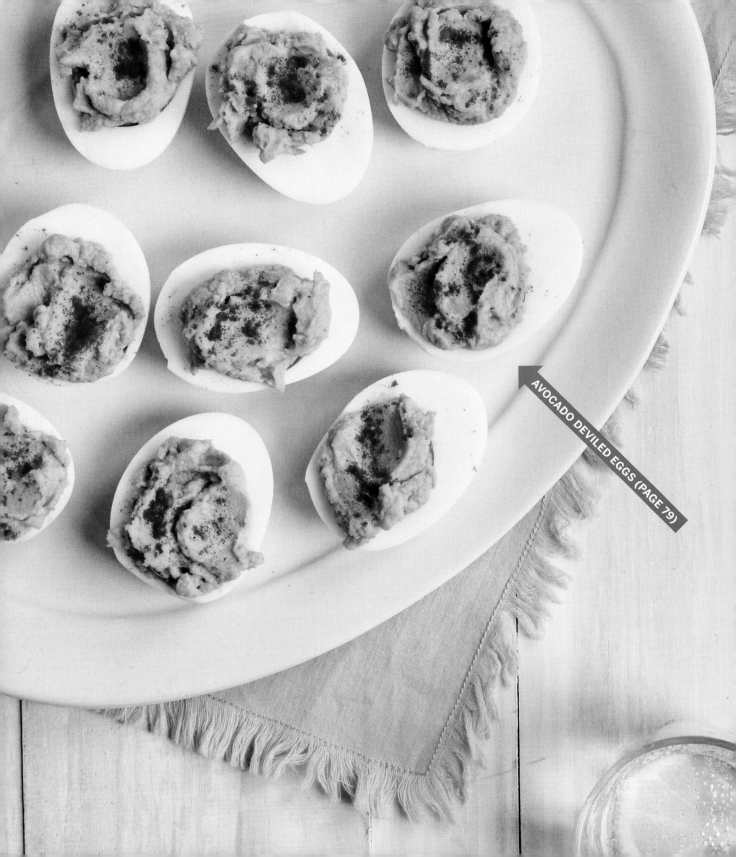

AVOCADO DEVILED EGGS (PAGE 79)

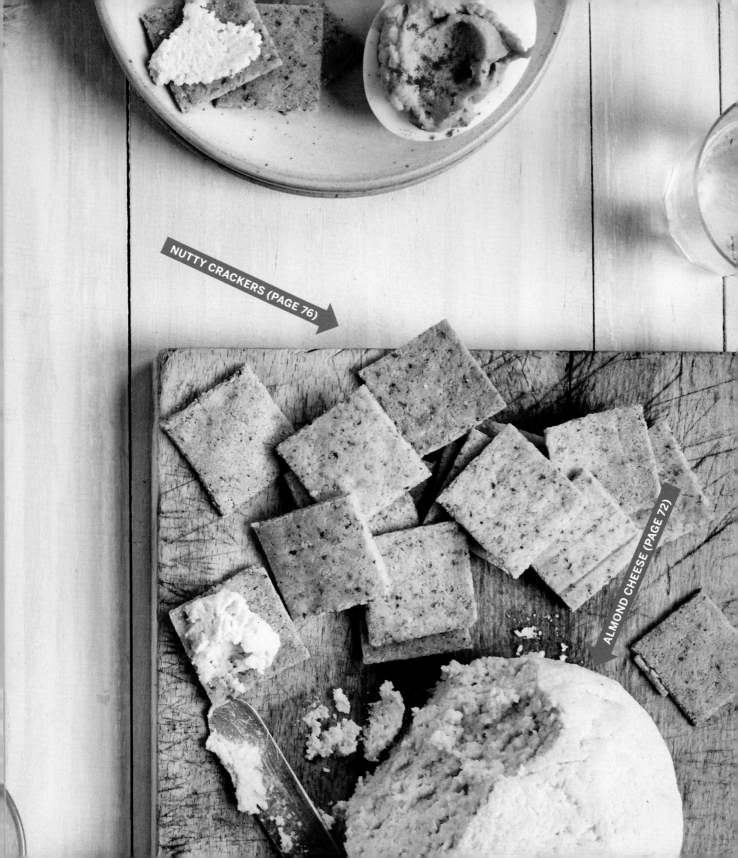

NUTTY CRACKERS (PAGE 76)

ALMOND CHEESE (PAGE 72)

NUTTY CRACKERS

DAIRY-FREE | EGG-FREE | PALEO

PREP TIME: 10 minutes
COOK TIME: 15 minutes
TOTAL TIME: 25 minutes
SERVINGS: 6

Craving something salty with a serious crunch factor? Try these low-carb crackers. They're way healthier than wheat-based ones because they contain omega-3s from flax and B vitamins from sunflower seeds.

1 cup blanched almond flour

2 tablespoons unsalted sunflower seeds

1 tablespoon flax meal

¾ teaspoon sea salt, plus extra for sprinkling

1 tablespoon coconut oil

Preheat the oven to 350°F.

Blend together the almond flour, sunflower seeds, flax meal, and sea salt in a bowl or food processor. If using a food processor, add 2 tablespoons water and the coconut oil and pulse until a dough forms. If blending by hand, stir 2 tablespoons water and the coconut oil into the dry ingredients to form a dough ball.

Place the dough ball on a sheet of parchment paper and press it flat. Cover with another sheet of parchment paper and roll the dough to a ⅛- to ¹⁄₁₆-inch thickness. Transfer to a cutting board, remove the top piece of parchment paper, and cut into 1-inch squares using a pizza cutter or knife. Sprinkle sea salt on top.

Transfer the sheet of parchment with the cut dough squares to a baking sheet and bake for 10 to 15 minutes, until the cracker edges are brown and crisp. Allow to cool on a rack, then separate the squares. Store in an airtight container for 3 to 5 days, depending on the humidity.

NOTES

Pair these with the Cheese Ball recipe (page 78) for an amazing keto appetizer! Or spread Almond Cheese (page 72) on them for a delicious dairy-free snack.

NUTRITIONAL DATA

151 calories, 13g fat, 291mg sodium, 2g fiber, 4g carbohydrates, 4g protein

2g net carbs, 6% carbs, 11% protein, 83% fat

STUFFED CUCUMBER SLICES

NUT-FREE | EGG-FREE

PREP TIME: 15 minutes
TOTAL TIME: 15 minutes
SERVINGS: 8

Cucumber slices topped with a mix of cream cheese and olives make for healthy finger food. Hosting a get-together at your house? Whip up this appetizer in no time.

2 large cucumbers, peeled and sliced crosswise into ¼-inch pieces

8 ounces cream cheese, softened

¼ cup whole pitted black olives, chopped

¼ cup pimento-stuffed olives, chopped

1 teaspoon onion powder

¼ teaspoon salt

NOTES

Just pimento-stuffed olives can be used if you don't like black olives.

NUTRITIONAL DATA

119 calories, 11g fat, 296mg sodium, 0g fiber, 3g carbohydrates, 2g protein

3g net carbs, 10% carbs, 7% protein, 83% fat

Use a melon baller or huller to remove the seeds from the center of the cucumber slices to make a small bowl-shaped cavity in each. Set aside.

In a medium bowl, blend together the cream cheese, black olives, pimento-stuffed olives, and onion powder in a medium bowl. Spoon the cream cheese mixture into the cavity in the center of the cucumber slices.

CHEESE BALL

PREP TIME: 15 minutes
TOTAL TIME: 15 minutes
SERVINGS: 16

You'll probably never hear a nutritionist say cheese balls are a superfood for health. But if you're burning fat for energy and need something super-low-carb in a pinch that's a cinch to make, this fits the bill. And it's sure to be a hit with family and friends.

½ cup chopped pecans

16 ounces cream cheese, softened

8 ounces cheddar cheese, grated

2 tablespoons mayonnaise

½ teaspoon onion powder

¼ teaspoon salt

Preheat the oven to 325°F. Spread the pecans in a single layer over a sheet pan and toast in the oven for about 5 minutes, then stir. Continue baking for another 5 minutes or until the pecans are fragrant, being careful not to burn. Let cool, then chop and place in a shallow bowl.

Add the cream cheese, cheddar cheese, mayonnaise, onion powder, and salt to a food processor and process until blended. Remove from the food processor and form the mixture into a ball. Roll the cheese ball in the chopped pecans. Chill for at least an hour before serving.

NOTES

Add chopped fresh parsley to the toasted pecans to give some color to the outside of the cheese ball. Or add the parsley to the cheese mixture for a little green inside.

NUTRITIONAL DATA

189 calories, 18g fat, 226mg sodium, 0g fiber, 1g carbohydrates, 5g protein

1g net carbs, 2% carbs, 11% protein, 87% fat

AVOCADO DEVILED EGGS

DAIRY-FREE | NUT-FREE | PALEO

PREP TIME: 15 minutes
TOTAL TIME: 15 minutes
SERVINGS: 6

They say the devil is in the details. So, does that mean the devil in deviled eggs is mayo? Well, if you can't stomach mayo, you'll be glad to know you can used mashed avocado as a velvety-smooth alternative.

6 large hard-cooked eggs

1 medium avocado

1 tablespoon lemon juice

⅛ teaspoon garlic powder

⅛ teaspoon salt

⅛ teaspoon paprika

Halve the eggs lengthwise. Remove the yolks from the whites and place in a mixing bowl.

Add the avocado, lemon juice, garlic powder, and salt to the egg yolks. Mash until the mixture is well combined. Pipe or spoon the mixture into the egg whites. Sprinkle paprika on top for garnish.

NOTES

Sliced jalapeños or olives can also be used to garnish the tops.

Chopped cooked pieces of bacon can be added to the avocado mixture for added flavor.

NUTRITIONAL DATA

117 calories, 9g fat, 113mg sodium, 2g fiber, 3g carbohydrates, 6g protein

1g net carbs, 4% carbs, 22% protein, 74% fat

SEASONED TORTILLA CHIPS

EGG-FREE

PREP TIME: 10 minutes
COOK TIME: 17 minutes
TOTAL TIME: 27 minutes
SERVINGS: 6

If you find most commercial tortilla chips taste way too salty, you'll enjoy these homemade spiced chips. They are savory plus high in protein, and are perfect for snacking or adding a little crunch to a salad.

1½ cups shredded mozzarella cheese

½ cup blanched almond flour

1 tablespoon flax meal

½ teaspoon onion powder

½ teaspoon ground cumin

¼ teaspoon salt

Preheat the oven to 375°F.

In a bowl, melt the mozzarella cheese in a microwave oven for 1 minute on high, stir, then heat for another 30 seconds or so until all the cheese is melted.

Stir in the almond flour, flax meal, onion powder, cumin, and salt. Roll the dough out on parchment paper or a silicone baking mat until it is very thin, ⅛ inch or less thick. Score into triangles using a pizza cutter or knife. (If using a silicone mat, use a duller knife so it doesn't cut the silicone.)

Bake for 10 to 15 minutes, until just golden brown.

Cool completely before serving. If not eating right away, store in an airtight container in the refrigerator for up to a week.

NOTES

The cumin and onion powder can be omitted for a plain chip to use for dips or for making loaded nachos.

NUTRITIONAL DATA

144 calories, 11g fat, 273mg sodium, 1g fiber, 3g carbohydrates, 8g protein

2g net carbs, 6% carbs, 23% protein, 71% fat

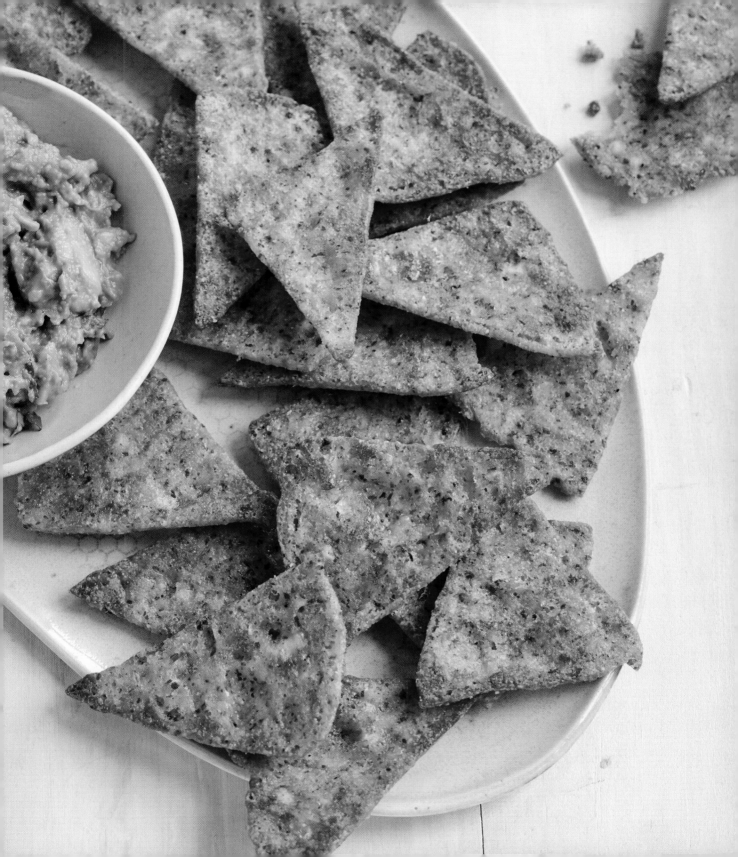

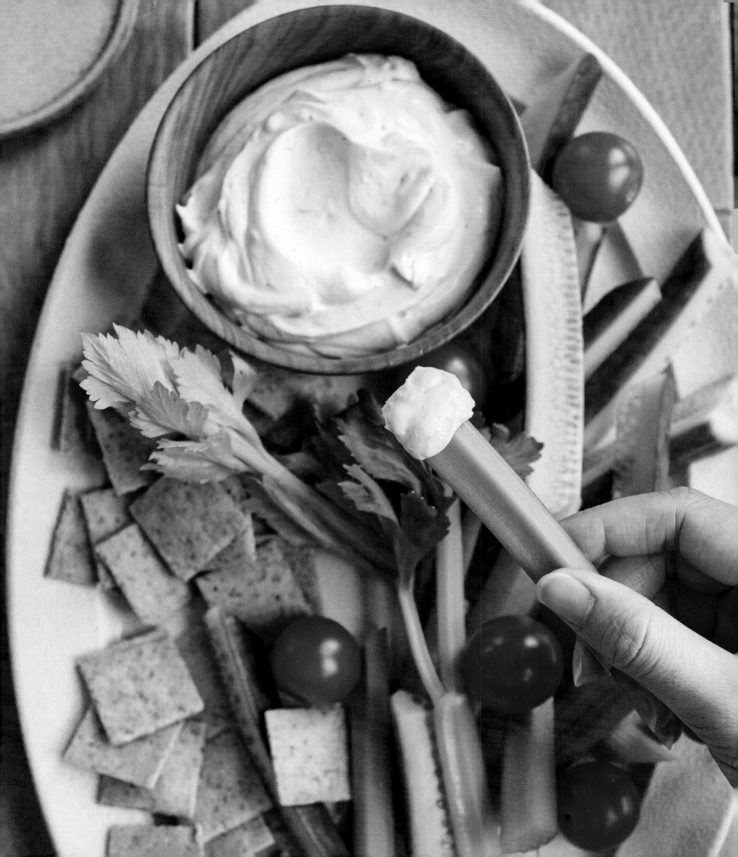

SOUR CREAM AND ONION DIP

NUT-FREE | EGG-FREE

PREP TIME: 5 minutes
TOTAL TIME: 5 minutes
SERVINGS: 8

A classic dip for dunking keto-friendly vegetables like cucumber slices and celery sticks, or to spread on low-carb crackers.

8 ounces cream cheese, softened

½ cup sour cream

1 teaspoon onion powder

½ teaspoon salt

¼ teaspoon dried dill

In a bowl, beat the cream cheese until smooth and fluffy. Blend in the sour cream, then mix in the onion powder, salt, and dill. Chill for an hour or two to allow the flavors to set in before serving.

NOTES

Plain almond milk yogurt and almond milk cream spread can be used to make this dairy-free.

NUTRITIONAL DATA

125 calories, 12g fat, 248mg sodium, 0g fiber, 1g carbohydrates, 2g protein

1g net carbs, 3% carbs, 7% protein, 90% fat

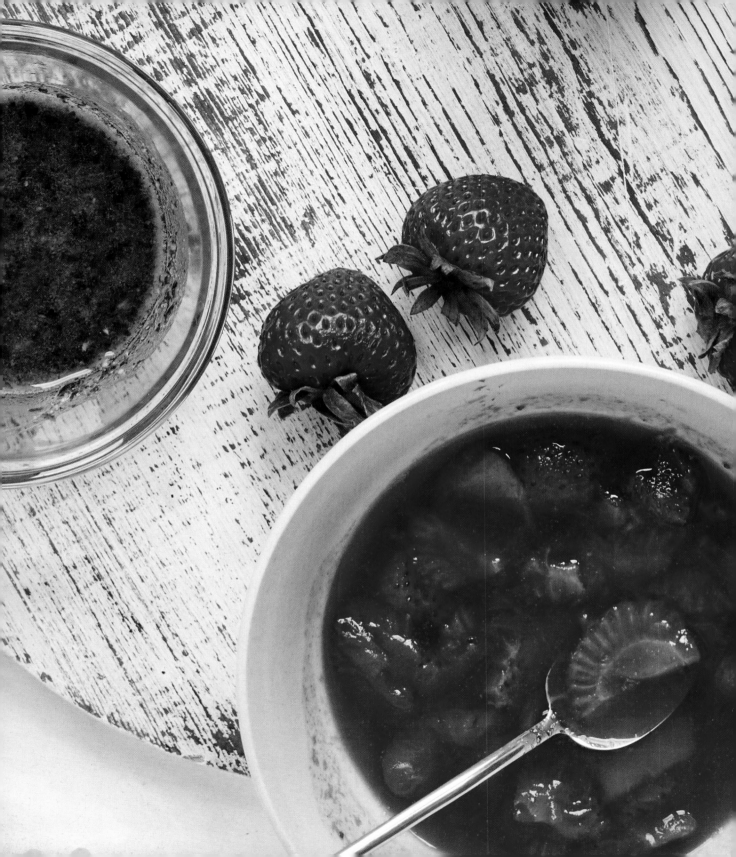

DRESSINGS AND SAUCES

Italian Dressing 86

Avocado Dressing 86

Chocolate Sauce 87

Strawberry Sauce 87

Maple Syrup 88

Avocado Mayonnaise 89

Cheese Sauce 92

Basil Pesto 92

Balsamic Vinaigrette 93

Blue Cheese Dressing 94

Low-Carb Ketchup 95

ITALIAN DRESSING

DAIRY-FREE | NUT-FREE | EGG-FREE | PALEO, AIP

PREP TIME: 5 minutes   TOTAL TIME: 5 minutes
SERVINGS: 4

A classic dressing that's got the perfect blend of acidity and sweetness. It's great for serving with tossed salads. The liquid stevia balances out the acidity of the vinegar, making it smooth to the palate.

3 tablespoons extra-virgin olive oil
¼ cup apple cider vinegar
20 drops liquid stevia extract
1 teaspoon Italian seasoning
Salt and black pepper (omit pepper for AIP)

In a jar or bowl, blend the olive oil, vinegar, stevia, and Italian seasoning together, season with salt and black pepper, and shake or stir before using. Store, covered, in the refrigerator up to 2 weeks and allow the dressing to come to room temperature before using.

NUTRITIONAL DATA

97 calories, 10g fat, 73mg sodium, 0g fiber, 0g carbohydrates, 0g protein

0g net carbs, 0% carbs, 0% protein, 100% fat

AVOCADO DRESSING

NUT-FREE | DAIRY-FREE | EGG-FREE | PALEO, AIP

PREP TIME: 5 minutes   TOTAL TIME: 5 minutes
SERVINGS: 6

Conventional creamy bottled dressings often contain added sugar and low-quality oil along with dairy, which I typically avoid. That's why I make my own creamy and thick dairy-free dressing with avocado.

1 medium avocado
½ cup Almond Milk (page 210) or coconut milk (for nut-free and AIP)
1 tablespoon lemon juice
2 tablespoons chopped fresh cilantro
1 clove garlic

Add the avocado, almond milk, lemon juice, cilantro, and garlic to a blender and blend until smooth. Store the leftovers in a sealed container in the refrigerator for up to a week.

NUTRITIONAL DATA

58 calories, 5g fat, 30mg sodium, 2g fiber, 3g carbohydrates, 1g protein

1g net carbs, 8% carbs, 8% protein, 85% fat

CHOCOLATE SAUCE

DAIRY-FREE | NUT-FREE | EGG-FREE

PREP TIME: 5 minutes	COOK TIME: 15 minutes
TOTAL TIME: 20 minutes	SERVINGS: 9

A dairy-free chocolate sauce that will satisfy any chocolate craving. Add a drizzle to vanilla ice cream, plain cake, or waffles. It's great for making chocolate almond milk, too.

½ cup unsweetened cocoa powder

¼ cup Swerve Confectioners sweetener

⅛ teaspoon sea salt

½ teaspoon vanilla extract

Whisk together 1 cup water, the cocoa powder, sweetener, and salt in a saucepan. Bring the mixture to a boil, then reduce the heat to low and simmer until the mixture thickens up a little, about 10 minutes. Remove from the heat and stir in the vanilla.

NOTES

You can add 1 tablespoon more sweetener at a time as needed, if you prefer it to be sweet.

NUTRITIONAL DATA

11 calories, 1g fat, 35mg sodium, 2g fiber, 3g carbohydrates, 0.4g erythritol, 1g protein

1g net carbs, 24% carbs, 24% protein, 53% fat

STRAWBERRY SAUCE

DAIRY-FREE | NUT-FREE | EGG-FREE

PREP TIME: 10 minutes	TOTAL TIME: 10 minutes
SERVINGS: 8	

Strawberry sauce drizzled over ice cream or cheesecake makes those desserts much more appealing, and with only 3 net grams of carbs, it won't have too much impact. It's also ideal for making strawberry shortcake.

1 pound strawberries, hulled and sliced

¼ cup monkfruit/erythritol granular sweetener

Place the strawberries in a medium saucepan. Add ½ cup water and the sweetener and gently stir to blend. Bring to a simmer and cook just until the berries have softened, about 10 minutes.

The sauce can be served warm or chilled. Store, covered, in the refrigerator for up to a week.

NUTRITIONAL DATA

18 calories, 1g fat, 1mg sodium, 1g fiber, 10g carbohydrates, 6g erythritol, 1g protein

3g net carbs, 48% carbs, 16% protein, 36% fat

MAPLE SYRUP

DAIRY-FREE | NUT-FREE | EGG-FREE

PREP TIME: 10 minutes
COOK TIME: 10 minutes
TOTAL TIME: 20 minutes
SERVINGS: 14 (2 tablespoons each)

There's no need to buy an expensive low-carb pancake syrup. It's easy to make at home using water, sweetener, and flavor extracts. And you can make it as thick or thin as you'd like! It goes wonderfully with my Almond Flour Pancakes (page 2) and Coconut Flour Waffles (page 17).

⅓ cup Swerve Confectioners sweetener

¼ teaspoon xanthan gum

¼ teaspoon salt

1 tablespoon maple extract

1 teaspoon vanilla extract

In a small saucepan, whisk together the Swerve, xanthan gum, and 2 cups water. Bring to a boil over medium-high heat, then reduce the heat to maintain a low simmer and cook for 5 minutes. Remove from the heat and stir in the maple extract and vanilla extract. Allow to cool before serving and store for up to 2 weeks in the refrigerator.

NOTES

The color of the syrup is a light amber. If you want a color closer to store-bought pancake syrup, you'll need to add in a little caramel coloring until the desired color is reached.

For a thicker syrup, add more xanthan gum a pinch at a time until the desired consistency is reached.

NUTRITIONAL DATA

1 calorie, 0g fat, 39mg sodium, 1g fiber, 6g carbohydrates, 5g erythritol, 0g protein

0g net carbs, 0% carbs, 0% protein, 0% fat

AVOCADO MAYONNAISE

PREP TIME: 5 minutes
COOK TIME: 5 minutes
TOTAL TIME: 10 minutes
SERVINGS: 12

DAIRY-FREE | NUT-FREE | PALEO

Avocado oil is a much healthier fat than the seed oils used in making conventional mayo. If you're looking to increase your healthy fat intake while enjoying a keto sandwich, this is the spread for you.

1 large egg yolk
1 tablespoon apple cider vinegar
¾ cup avocado oil
⅛ teaspoon salt

Whisk together the egg yolk and vinegar in a small pot. Set over low heat and cook, whisking constantly, until the mixture is frothy and thick, being careful not to cook the egg into solid bits, about 5 minutes.

Remove from the heat, allow to cool slightly, then slowly whisk in the oil and salt until the dressing becomes creamy. Store, covered, in the refrigerator for 1 to 2 weeks.

NOTES

An immersion blender works best to incorporate the oil.

If you feel the yolks are safe to be eaten raw, the cooking step can be skipped.

NUTRITIONAL DATA

126 calories, 14g fat, 25mg sodium, 0g fiber, 0g carbohydrates, 1g protein

0g net carbs, 0% carbs, 3% protein, 97% fat

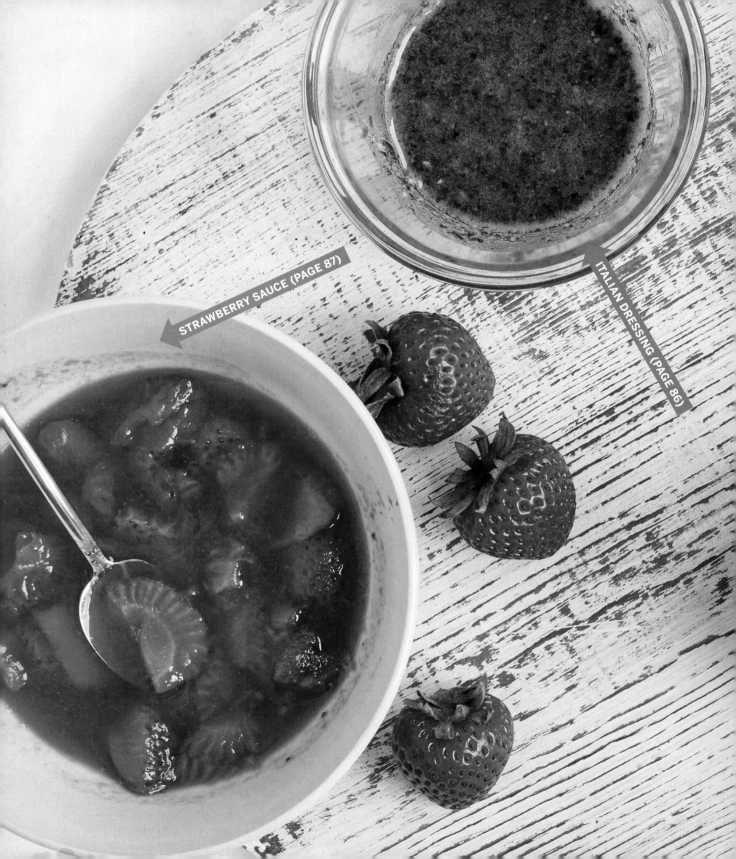

STRAWBERRY SAUCE (PAGE 87)

ITALIAN DRESSING (PAGE 86)

AVOCADO DRESSING (PAGE 86)

CHEESE SAUCE (PAGE 92)

BALSAMIC VINAIGRETTE (PAGE 93)

CHEESE SAUCE

NUT-FREE | EGG-FREE

PREP TIME: 5 minutes COOK TIME: 10 minutes
TOTAL TIME: 15 minutes SERVINGS: 8

Almost anything tastes better dipped in cheese, especially steamed veggies. The kids may never complain about eating their vegetables again!

4 ounces cheddar cheese, grated

1 cup heavy cream

2 teaspoons Dijon mustard

Combine the cheddar cheese, heavy cream, and mustard in a medium saucepan over medium heat. Cook, stirring, until all of the cheese is melted. Use immediately. If the sauce cools, it will need to be warmed on the stovetop or in the microwave.

NUTRITIONAL DATA

165 calories, 15g fat, 242mg sodium, 1g fiber, 1g carbohydrates, 6g protein

0g net carbs, 0% carbs, 15% protein, 85% fat

BASIL PESTO

DAIRY-FREE | EGG-FREE | PALEO

PREP TIME: 5 minutes COOK TIME: 15 minutes
TOTAL TIME: 20 minutes SERVINGS: 6

Who says you have to travel to Italy to learn the art of making great pesto? This recipe is easy to make and works as a dip, a spread, or a topping for grilled meats.

3 tablespoons pecans

2 cups fresh basil leaves

¼ cup extra-virgin olive oil

2 teaspoons minced garlic

Preheat the oven to 325°F. Spread the pecans in a single layer over a sheet pan and toast in the oven for 5 minutes, then stir and bake for another 5 minutes or until fragrant. Let cool completely.

After the pecans have cooled, add them to a food processor or blender with the basil leaves, olive oil, and garlic. Puree until smooth.

NUTRITIONAL DATA

117 calories, 13g fat, 1mg sodium, 1g fiber, 1g carbohydrates, 1g protein

0g net carbs, 0% carbs, 17% protein, 83% fat

BALSAMIC VINAIGRETTE

NUT-FREE | DAIRY-FREE | EGG-FREE | PALEO

PREP TIME: 5 minutes
TOTAL TIME: 5 minutes
SERVINGS: 12

Another classic dressing you can easily make at home. This flavorful vinaigrette is the perfect balance of subtly sweet and tart.

1 cup extra-virgin olive oil

⅓ cup balsamic vinegar

1 clove garlic, minced

1 tablespoon Dijon mustard

1 teaspoon salt

½ teaspoon black pepper

Add the olive oil, balsamic vinegar, garlic, Dijon mustard, salt, and black pepper to a blender and blend until well combined. Transfer to an airtight container. Store, covered, in the refrigerator for up to 2 weeks. Allow to come to room temperature before using.

NOTES

Best if allowed to sit for an hour before using to infuse the flavors.

NUTRITIONAL DATA

167 calories, 18g fat, 210mg sodium, 1g fiber, 1g carbohydrates, 1g protein

0g net carbs, 0% carbs, 2% protein, 98% fat

BLUE CHEESE DRESSING

NUT-FREE

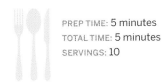

PREP TIME: 5 minutes
TOTAL TIME: 5 minutes
SERVINGS: 10

A creamy yet tangy dressing that's full of blue cheese crumbles. It's a classic recipe to top any green leaf salad.

⅓ cup sour cream

½ cup mayonnaise

5 ounces blue cheese, crumbled

2 tablespoons lemon juice

¼ teaspoon garlic powder

Salt and black pepper

Blend the sour cream, mayonnaise, blue cheese, lemon juice, garlic powder, and salt and black pepper to taste together in a medium bowl. Adjust the seasonings if needed.

Chill for at least 2 hours to allow the flavors to combine before serving.

NOTES

The cheese can be broken into smaller pieces for a less chunky dressing.

NUTRITIONAL DATA

82 calories, 7g fat, 292mg sodium, 0g fiber, 1g carbohydrates, 4g protein

1g net carbs, 5% carbs, 19% protein, 76% fat

LOW-CARB KETCHUP

DAIRY-FREE | NUT-FREE | EGG-FREE | PALEO

PREP TIME: 10 minutes
COOK TIME: 25 minutes
TOTAL TIME: 35 minutes
SERVINGS: 20 (about 2 tablespoons each)

It can be challenging to find a commercially prepared ketchup without added sugar. But making your own is always an option and is extremely easy to do. Just be sure to make only what you need or freeze any extra for long-term storage.

1 (28-ounce) can whole skinned and seeded tomatoes, drained

¼ cup tomato paste

1 tablespoon apple cider vinegar

2 teaspoons onion powder

1 teaspoon garlic powder

1 teaspoon salt

15 to 30 drops stevia liquid extract (optional)

Add the canned tomatoes, tomato paste, vinegar, onion powder, garlic powder, and salt to a medium saucepan. Heat over medium-low heat, stirring frequently, for 12 to 15 minutes.

Remove from the heat. Puree using an immersion blender (or let cool briefly and transfer to a regular blender). Continue to cook over medium-low heat, stirring occasionally, until the sauce thickens, another 8 to 10 minutes. If needed, add sweetener to taste.

Cool completely, then transfer to an airtight container and store in the refrigerator for up to 2 weeks.

NOTES

For longer storage, the ketchup can be frozen for up to 3 months.

Puree in a blender after cooking is complete for a smoother consistency.

NUTRITIONAL DATA

11 calories, 1g fat, 199mg sodium, 1g fiber, 2g carbohydrates, 1g protein

1g net carbs, 24% carbs, 24% protein, 52% fat

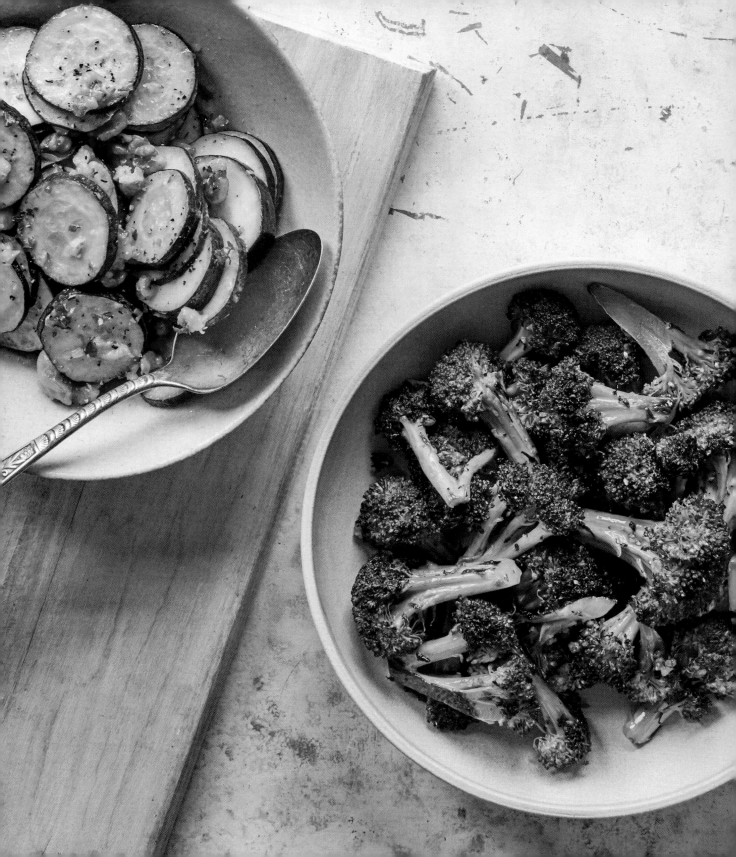

SIDE DISHES

Fried Spinach with Mushrooms 98

Stir-Fried Squash and Pepper 101

Fried Cabbage with Bacon 102

Wilted Lettuce with Bacon 104

Cauliflower Mash 105

Turnip Fries 106

Mushrooms Provençale 107

Sautéed Celery 107

Pork Fried Rice 109

Roasted Broccoli 110

Almond Asparagus 111

Creamed Spinach 114

Sautéed Red Cabbage 114

Walnut Zucchini 115

FRIED SPINACH WITH MUSHROOMS

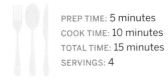

PREP TIME: 5 minutes
COOK TIME: 10 minutes
TOTAL TIME: 15 minutes
SERVINGS: 4

DAIRY-FREE | NUT-FREE | EGG-FREE | PALEO, AIP

When you want to get more veggies in your diet, this sautéed spinach with mushrooms is the perfect companion to grilled meats. Or serve it to your vegetarian friends.

2 tablespoons extra-virgin olive oil

8 ounces white button or baby bella mushrooms, sliced

2 cloves garlic, minced

15 cups (10 ounces) baby spinach leaves

Salt and black pepper (omit pepper for AIP)

Heat the oil in a skillet over medium-high heat. Add the mushrooms and garlic and cook, stirring, until the garlic is fragrant and the mushrooms are soft, about 5 minutes. Add the spinach and stir constantly until the spinach has wilted. Remove from the heat and season with salt and black pepper to taste.

NOTES

Butter can be used in place of olive oil for a buttery flavor if dairy isn't an issue.

NUTRITIONAL DATA

92 calories, 7g fat, 59mg sodium, 2g fiber, 4g carbohydrates, 3g protein

2g net carbs, 10% carbs, 14% protein, 76% fat

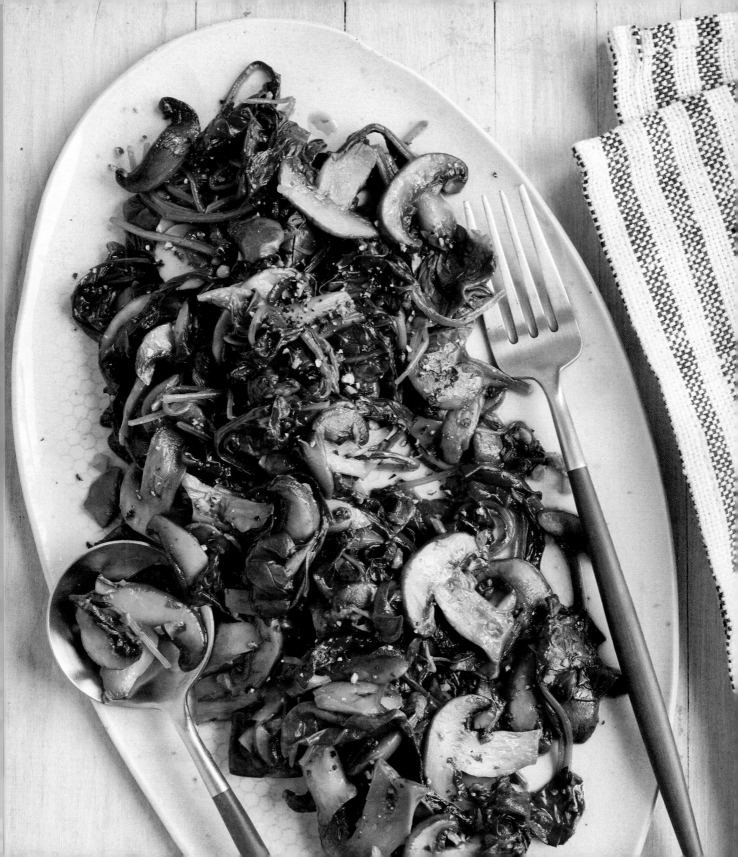

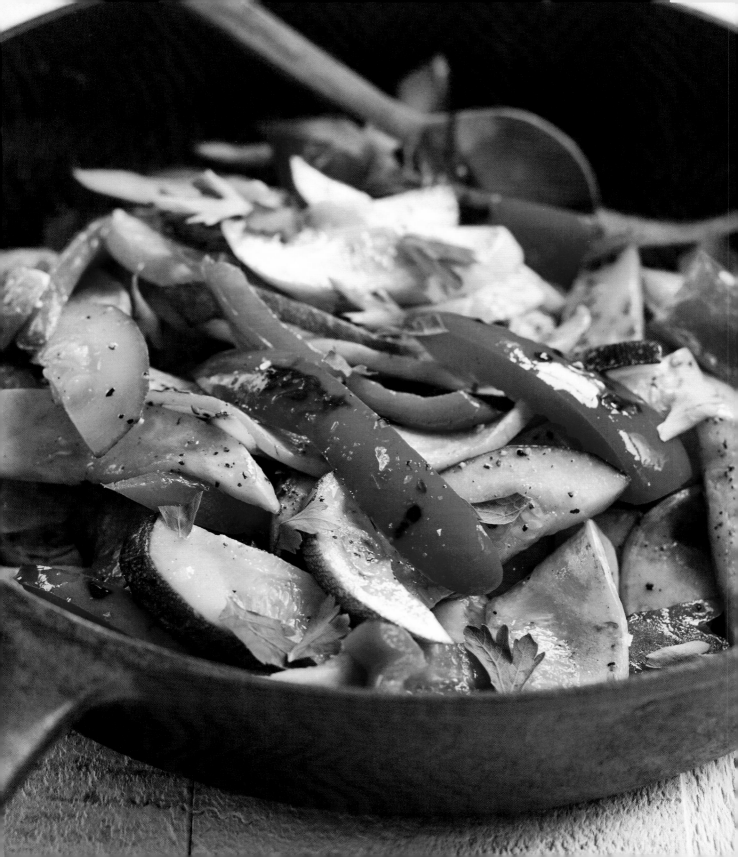

STIR-FRIED SQUASH AND PEPPER

PREP TIME: 10 minutes
COOK TIME: 9 minutes
TOTAL TIME: 19 minutes
SERVINGS: 6

DAIRY-FREE | NUT-FREE | EGG-FREE | PALEO

A colorful side dish with zucchini, yellow squash, and red pepper, it's a great combination of summer vegetables!

2 medium zucchini

2 medium yellow squash

1 red bell pepper, seeded

3 tablespoons extra-virgin olive oil

Salt and black pepper

1 tablespoon chopped fresh parsley (optional), for garnish

Cut the zucchini, squash, and bell pepper into thin strips of similar size.

Heat the oil in a large skillet over medium heat and add the sliced zucchini and yellow squash. Cook, stirring often, until the vegetables are tender, 3 to 4 minutes. Add the red pepper slices and cook, stirring, until all the vegetables are tender, about 3 minutes longer.

Add salt and black pepper to taste. Garnish with the parsley, if desired.

NOTES

Green peppers have fewer carbs than red and can be used instead, but the dish won't be as colorful.

NUTRITIONAL DATA

89 calories, 7g fat, 55mg sodium, 1g fiber, 5g carbohydrates, 1g protein

4g net carbs, 18% carbs, 13% protein, 69% fat

FRIED CABBAGE WITH BACON

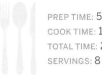

PREP TIME: 5 minutes
COOK TIME: 15 minutes
TOTAL TIME: 20 minutes
SERVINGS: 8

DAIRY-FREE | NUT-FREE | EGG-FREE | PALEO, AIP IF MODIFIED

Frying cabbage in bacon fat makes it so tasty, especially when pieces of bacon are added into the mix. This is sure to become a regular dish you'll enjoy over and over.

12 slices bacon, chopped

½ cup minced onion

2 cloves garlic

1 medium head cabbage, shredded

½ teaspoon salt

⅛ teaspoon black pepper (omit for AIP)

⅛ teaspoon paprika (omit for AIP)

Add the bacon, onion, and garlic to a large skillet over medium heat and cook, stirring, until the onion is tender and the bacon is cooked, 5 to 7 minutes.

Stir in the shredded cabbage. Season with the salt, black pepper, and paprika. Continue cooking, stirring occasionally, until the cabbage is tender, 6 to 8 minutes more.

NOTES

If using precooked bacon, the cabbage can be fried in melted butter or coconut oil instead of the bacon fat.

NUTRITIONAL DATA

171 calories, 13g fat, 530mg sodium, 3g fiber, 8g carbohydrates, 5g protein

5g net carbs, 13% carbs, 13% protein, 75% fat

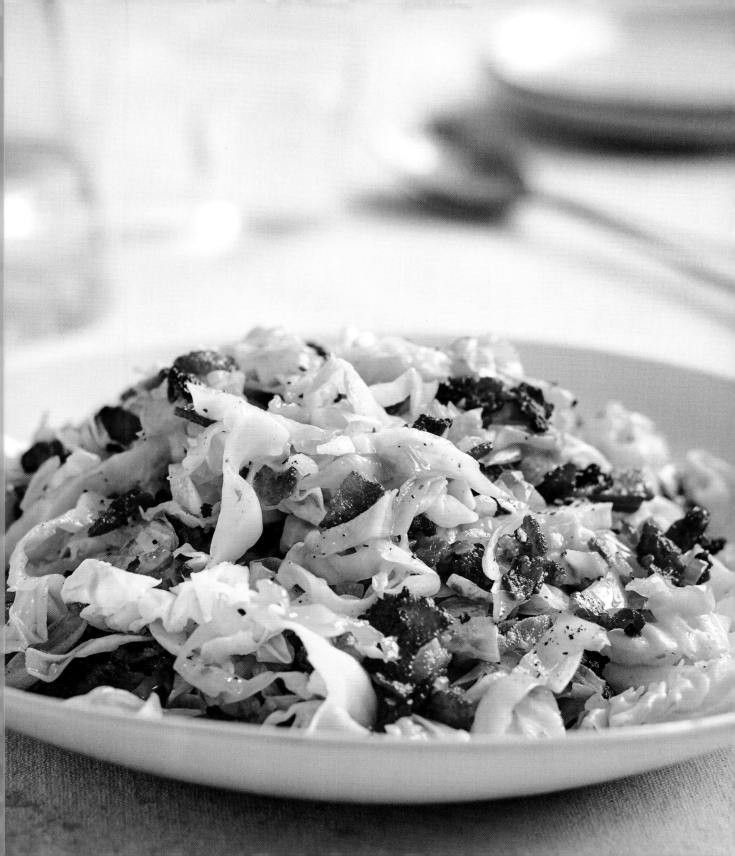

WILTED LETTUCE WITH BACON

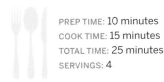

PREP TIME: 10 minutes
COOK TIME: 15 minutes
TOTAL TIME: 25 minutes
SERVINGS: 4

DAIRY-FREE | NUT-FREE | EGG-FREE | PALEO, AIP

Wilted lettuce may not sound like the most appetizing thing to eat, but you're in for a surprise when wilted romaine pairs with fried bacon along with a sweet and tangy vinegar sauce.

8 slices bacon, chopped

½ cup distilled white vinegar

1 tablespoon lemon juice

10 drops liquid stevia extract, or equivalent sweetener

8 cups chopped romaine lettuce

Add the bacon to a large pot over medium-high heat and cook, stirring occasionally, until crisp, 5 to 7 minutes. Stir in the vinegar, lemon juice, and sweetener until well blended. Add the lettuce and cook, stirring, until it's wilted, 1 to 2 minutes. Serve warm.

NOTES

A teaspoon or two of Dijon mustard tastes great added to the sauce.

NUTRITIONAL DATA

206 calories, 17g fat, 299mg sodium, 1g fiber, 6g carbohydrates, 6g protein

5g net carbs, 10% carbs, 12% protein, 78% fat

CAULIFLOWER MASH

NUT-FREE | EGG-FREE

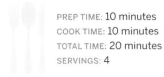

PREP TIME: 10 minutes
COOK TIME: 10 minutes
TOTAL TIME: 20 minutes
SERVINGS: 4

Want to know the secret for never missing mashed potatoes again? Perfect the art of making cauliflower mash. All it takes is a few steps, and adding cheese to the mashed cooked vegetable gives it a thicker texture like that of mashed potatoes.

1 medium head cauliflower (about 1 pound), chopped

2 ounces cream cheese

2 tablespoons grated Parmesan cheese

1 tablespoon butter

½ teaspoon salt

⅛ teaspoon black pepper

1 tablespoon sliced fresh chives (optional), for garnish

Steam the cauliflower until it's very soft, about 10 minutes.

Add the cooked cauliflower with the cream cheese, Parmesan cheese, butter, salt, and black pepper to a blender or food processor (or combine them in a large bowl and use an electric mixer). Blend until smooth and the cauliflower is well mashed. Garnish with chives, if desired.

NOTES

Add 1 clove roasted garlic for added flavor.

Use almond milk cream cheese spread, butter-flavored coconut oil, and nutritional yeast in place of the cheeses and butter for a dairy-free version.

NUTRITIONAL DATA

119 calories, 8g fat, 299mg sodium, 2g fiber, 7g carbohydrates, 4g protein

5g net carbs, 19% carbs, 15% protein, 67% fat

TURNIP FRIES

DAIRY-FREE | NUT-FREE | EGG-FREE | PALEO

PREP TIME: 10 minutes
COOK TIME: 30 minutes
TOTAL TIME: 40 minutes
SERVINGS: 8

When you're craving french fries, can turnips do the trick? While I can't promise you'll think they taste exactly like fast-food fries, they do provide a close-enough healthy alternative. Just eat a small serving size to keep carbs down.

2 pounds turnips (4 medium purple-topped)

2 tablespoons extra-virgin olive oil

1 teaspoon ground cumin

½ teaspoon Cajun seasoning

¼ teaspoon sea salt, plus more as needed

¼ teaspoon garlic powder

Preheat the oven to 425°F. Oil a sheet pan.

Peel the turnips and slice into french fry–shaped pieces. Place the cut turnips into a large bowl. Coat with the olive oil. Sprinkle with the cumin, Cajun seasoning, salt, and garlic powder and toss to blend.

Spread the turnip fries evenly over the prepared sheet pan. Bake for 20 to 30 minutes.

Sprinkle the fries with additional salt to taste.

NOTES

Regular or smoked paprika can be used in place of the Cajun seasoning. Stick to a small half-turnip-size serving, as the carbs can add up quickly if too many are eaten.

NUTRITIONAL DATA

64 calories, 3g fat, 149mg sodium, 2g fiber, 7g carbohydrates, 1g protein

5g net carbs, 39% carbs, 8% protein, 53% fat

MUSHROOMS PROVENÇALE

NUT-FREE | EGG-FREE

PREP TIME: 5 minutes   COOK TIME: 7 minutes
TOTAL TIME: 12 minutes   SERVINGS: 4

This classic French dish with buttery sautéed mushrooms will take your steak to the next level. Prepare it while the steak is cooking.

2 tablespoons butter

8 ounces baby bella mushrooms, sliced

1 teaspoon chopped fresh chives

1 clove garlic, minced

1 teaspoon lemon juice

¼ teaspoon salt

Black pepper

Melt the butter in a skillet over medium-high heat. Add the mushrooms and cook, stirring occasionally, until softened a bit, 4 to 5 minutes. Add the chives, garlic, lemon juice, salt, and black pepper and cook, stirring, for about 2 minutes more. Adjust the seasonings if needed.

NOTES

Can be garnished with chopped fresh parsley.

NUTRITIONAL DATA

64 calories, 5g fat, 270mg sodium, 0g fiber, 2g carbohydrates, 1g protein

2g net carbs, 14% carbs, 7% protein, 79% fat

SAUTÉED CELERY

DAIRY-FREE | NUT-FREE | EGG-FREE | PALEO, AIP

PREP TIME: 10 minutes   COOK TIME: 7 minutes
TOTAL TIME: 17 minutes   SERVINGS: 4

Celery isn't a veggie that most people think about sautéing; however, cooking it removes some of the bitter taste. Plus, it softens it up a bit without losing all the crunch. You can add it to a salad or soup or a healthy low-carb stir-fry. I like to season it with thyme to enhance the flavor.

2 tablespoons avocado oil or butter

6 stalks celery, thinly sliced diagonally (about 2 cups)

½ teaspoon fresh thyme leaves

½ teaspoon salt

⅛ teaspoon black pepper (omit for AIP)

In a large skillet over medium heat, heat the oil, then add the celery, thyme, salt, and black pepper. Cook, stirring occasionally, until the celery is crisp-tender, about 5 minutes.

NOTES

Chopped onions can be added for additional flavor.

NUTRITIONAL DATA

70 calories, 7g fat, 331mg sodium, 0g fiber, 1g carbohydrates, 0g protein

1g net carbs, 6% carbs, 0% protein, 94% fat

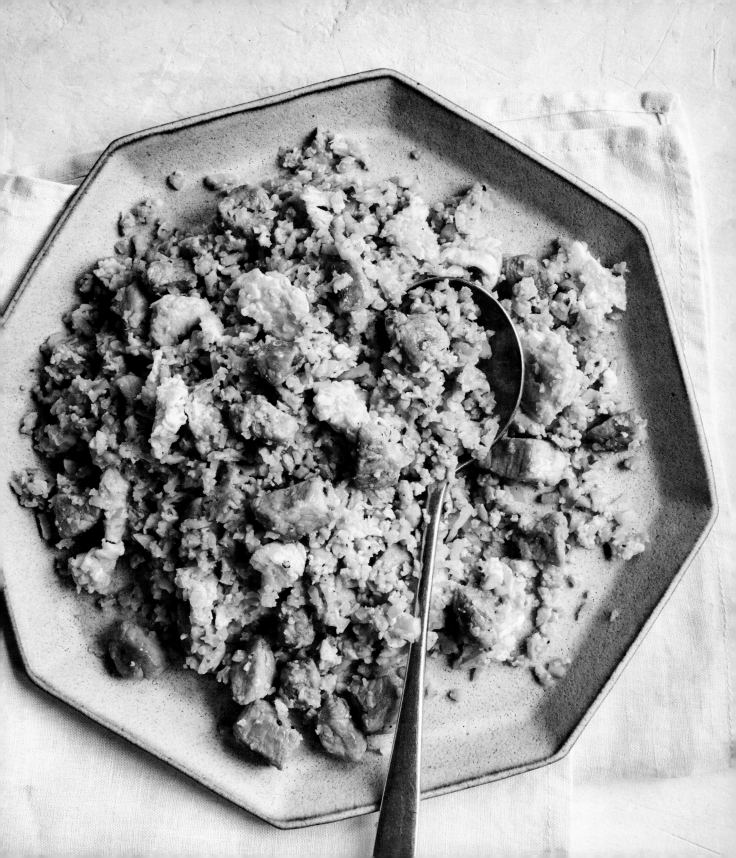

PORK FRIED RICE

DAIRY-FREE | NUT-FREE | PALEO

PREP TIME: 5 minutes
COOK TIME: 10 minutes
TOTAL TIME: 15 minutes
SERVINGS: 4

A classic dish made without all the traditional carbs! When you stir-fry riced cauliflower and add coconut aminos, scrambled eggs, and a little meat, you'll think you're eating Chinese fast food.

3 tablespoons extra-virgin olive oil

3 cloves garlic, minced

3 cups riced cauliflower, cooked

3 large eggs, beaten

½ cup diced cooked pork

1 tablespoon coconut aminos

Heat the oil over medium-high heat in a large skillet or wok. Add the garlic and cook, stirring, until fragrant, 30 seconds to a minute. Stir the riced cauliflower into the oil and garlic, then push to the side.

Pour the beaten eggs into the pan in the opened area and scramble for 2 to 3 minutes. Stir the scrambled cooked eggs into the riced cauliflower and then stir in the pork.

Mix in the coconut aminos and stir over medium heat until all is well heated, 1 to 2 minutes.

NOTES

Raw bacon pieces can be subbed for cooked pork. Just fry them in the pan first and use the bacon grease to stir-fry instead of adding oil.

One pound of cooked ground pork can be used in place of the diced cooked pork. Add it after the oil is hot and stir with a wooden spoon until cooked through.

NUTRITIONAL DATA
203 calories, 16g fat, 333mg sodium, 1g fiber, 4g carbohydrates, 10g protein

3g net carbs, 6% carbs, 20% protein, 73% fat

HOW TO COOK CAULIFLOWER RICE

To make cauliflower rice from scratch, shred a whole head of cauliflower in a food processor with the grating blade. Transfer the shredded cauliflower to a microwave-safe glass dish, cover with a lid, and microwave on high for 5 minutes.

ROASTED BROCCOLI

DAIRY-FREE | NUT-FREE | EGG-FREE | PALEO, AIP

PREP TIME: 5 minutes
COOK TIME: 15 minutes
TOTAL TIME: 20 minutes
SERVINGS: 4

Baking broccoli on a sheet pan releases some of the natural vegetable sugar to give it a slightly sweeter taste than when you steam it. Many prefer the taste over steaming or stir-frying.

12 ounces broccoli, cut into florets

2 tablespoons extra-virgin olive oil

2 cloves garlic, minced

½ teaspoon salt

Preheat the oven to 425°F.

Combine the broccoli, olive oil, garlic, and salt together and then spread over a rimmed baking sheet. Bake for 10 to 15 minutes, until the broccoli is tender and starting to brown. Toss the broccoli at least once during the middle of the baking time for even cooking.

NOTES

Be sure not to overlap the broccoli florets. They should be roasted in a single layer.

It's best to cut the florets in even pieces so the smaller pieces don't burn before the larger ones are done roasting.

NUTRITIONAL DATA

93 calories, 7g fat, 319mg sodium, 2g fiber, 6g carbohydrates, 2g protein

4g net carbs, 18% carbs, 9% protein, 72% fat

ALMOND ASPARAGUS

EGG-FREE

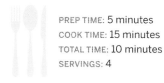
PREP TIME: 5 minutes
COOK TIME: 15 minutes
TOTAL TIME: 10 minutes
SERVINGS: 4

A double dose of crunch! Tossing in a few slivered almonds adds a nutty taste to garlic butter asparagus.

4 tablespoons butter

1 pound fresh asparagus

½ cup slivered almonds

3 cloves garlic, thinly sliced

1 tablespoon lemon juice

Salt and black pepper

Melt the butter in a large skillet over medium-high heat. Add the asparagus, almonds, and garlic and cook, stirring occasionally, for 3 to 5 minutes.

Reduce the heat to medium, cover, and cook until the asparagus is crisp-tender, about 2 minutes. Season with the lemon juice and salt and black pepper to taste.

NOTES

Use butter-flavored coconut oil to make this dairy-free.

NUTRITIONAL DATA

206 calories, 18g fat, 249mg sodium, 4g fiber, 8g carbohydrates, 5g protein

4g net carbs, 8% carbs, 10% protein, 82% fat

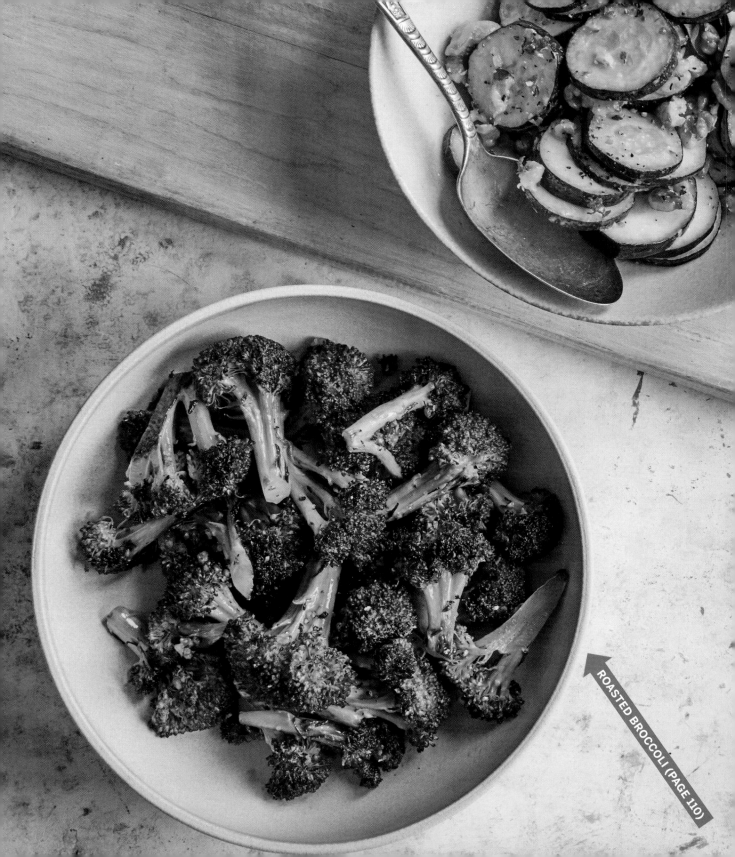

ROASTED BROCCOLI (PAGE 110)

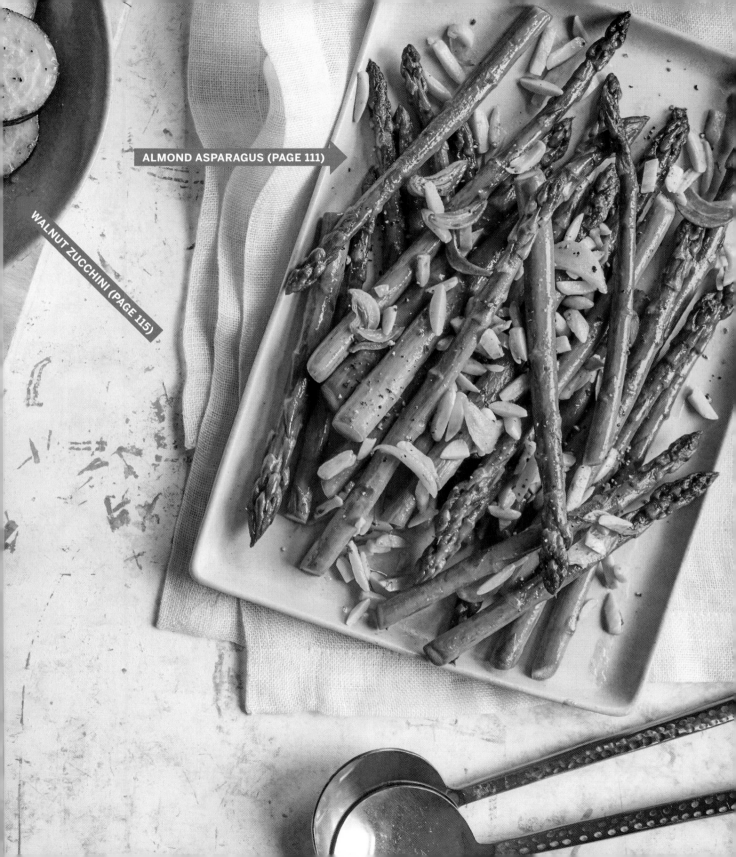

ALMOND ASPARAGUS (PAGE 111)

WALNUT ZUCCHINI (PAGE 115)

CREAMED SPINACH

NUT-FREE | EGG-FREE

PREP TIME: 5 minutes	COOK TIME: 35 minutes
TOTAL TIME: 40 minutes	SERVINGS: 4

Get them to eat their spinach by combining it with a cheesy cream sauce! Creamed spinach makes an excellent holiday side dish too.

10 ounces frozen spinach

4 ounces cream cheese, softened

2 tablespoons butter, softened

½ cup heavy cream

¼ cup grated Parmesan cheese

Cook the spinach in a pot according to the package instructions—about 6 minutes in a small amount of boiling water, covered. Drain and return the spinach to the pot.

Add the cream cheese, butter, heavy cream, and Parmesan cheese to the pot with the spinach. Heat over medium heat until the cheese is melted and well blended with the spinach, 3 to 5 minutes.

NOTES

If the cheese sauce becomes too thick, a little water can be added to thin it out after the cheese has melted.

NUTRITIONAL DATA

168 calories, 16g fat, 193mg sodium, 2g fiber, 4g carbohydrates, 4g protein

2g net carbs, 3% carbs, 7% protein, 90% fat

SAUTÉED RED CABBAGE

DAIRY-FREE | NUT-FREE | EGG-FREE | PALEO, AIP

PREP TIME: 10 minutes	COOK TIME: 15 minutes
TOTAL TIME: 25 minutes	SERVINGS: 6

Red cabbage is enjoying elite status as a superfood, and deservedly so. It may help lower blood pressure and blood sugar. Preserve the benefits of it and bring out the taste by sautéing in oil with a tangy vinegar seasoning.

2 tablespoons extra-virgin olive oil

½ red cabbage, thinly sliced and chopped into bite-size pieces

⅓ cup apple cider vinegar

5 drops stevia liquid extract

1 teaspoon yellow mustard seed (omit for AIP)

Salt

Heat the oil in a skillet over medium-high heat. Add the cabbage and cook, stirring, until it wilts, 3 to 5 minutes. Stir in the vinegar and stevia. Stir in the mustard seed and add salt to taste.

Reduce the heat slightly and let the cabbage cook, stirring occasionally, for another 10 minutes.

NUTRITIONAL DATA

68 calories, 4g fat, 116mg sodium, 1g fiber, 5g carbohydrates, 1g protein

4g net carbs, 29% carbs, 7% protein, 64% fat

WALNUT ZUCCHINI

EGG-FREE

PREP TIME: 10 minutes
COOK TIME: 10 minutes
TOTAL TIME: 20 minutes
SERVINGS: 4

Another pairing of crunchy nuts and veggies. I like that walnuts are high in ALA omega-3 fatty acid and antioxidants, while zucchini is a good source of potassium.

3 tablespoons butter

3 cloves garlic, chopped

2 medium zucchini, sliced

¼ cup chopped walnuts

¼ teaspoon chopped fresh oregano

Salt and black pepper

Melt the butter in a skillet over medium heat. Add the garlic and cook, stirring, until fragrant, 30 seconds to 1 minute. Stir in the zucchini, walnuts, and oregano. Cover and cook for 5 minutes. Uncover and cook, stirring, until the zucchini is tender, 3 to 4 minutes more. Season with salt and black pepper to taste.

NOTES

Add sliced red bell pepper with the zucchini for color.

Use olive oil or butter-flavored coconut oil to make this dairy-free.

NUTRITIONAL DATA

143 calories, 13g fat, 83mg sodium, 1g fiber, 4g carbohydrates, 2g protein

3g net carbs, 9% carbs, 6% protein, 85% fat

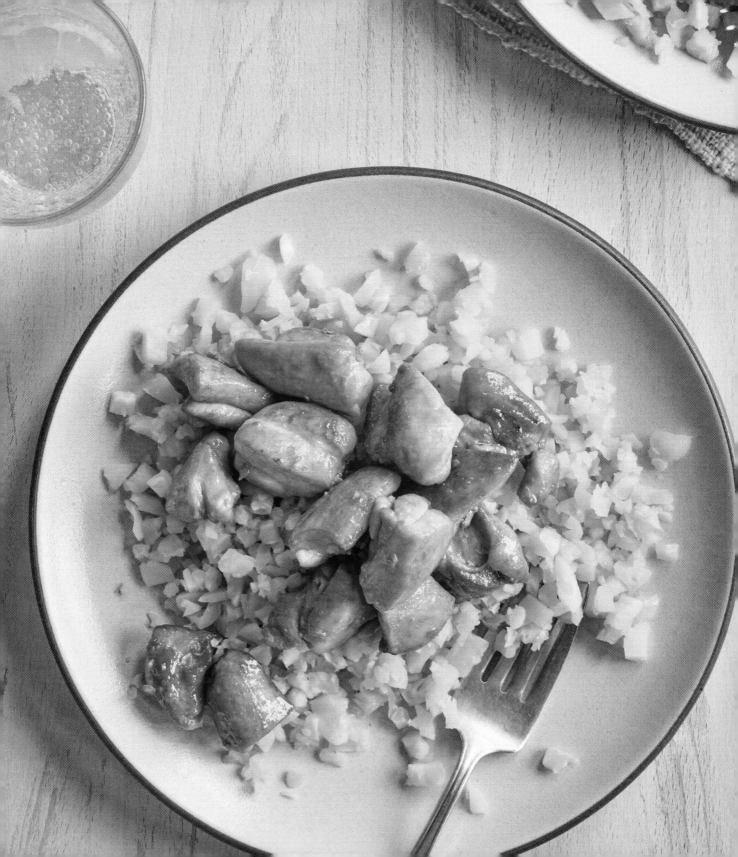

MAIN DISHES: POULTRY AND PORK

Roasted Chicken 118

Garlic-Lemon Chicken 120

Chicken-Broccoli Casserole 121

Broccoli and Cheese Stuffed Chicken 123

Baked Chicken Thighs 124

Curried Chicken 127

Marinated Turkey Tenderloins 128

Smothered Pork Chops 129

Filipino Chicken Adobo 130

Ham and Collard Greens 133

Egg Roll in a Bowl 134

Pork Loin Roast 136

Chicken with Spinach and Tomato 137

Quick "Breaded" Pork 139

ROASTED CHICKEN

DAIRY-FREE | NUT-FREE | EGG-FREE | PALEO, AIP

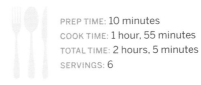

PREP TIME: 10 minutes
COOK TIME: 1 hour, 55 minutes
TOTAL TIME: 2 hours, 5 minutes
SERVINGS: 6

Go ahead and stuff it! Take roast chicken to a whole other level by stuffing it with lemon and savory herbs. Transform plain chicken into a succulent, juicy, more flavorful, and tender entrée. It's way easier than it sounds.

4- to 5-pound whole chicken

1 lemon, sliced

1 bunch fresh parsley

4 sprigs fresh thyme

2 cloves garlic

Salt and black pepper (omit pepper for AIP)

Preheat the oven to 450°F.

Stuff the chicken with the lemon slices, parsley, and thyme. Peel the garlic and either put it in the cavity with the herbs, or cut slits in the skin and tuck the pieces of garlic into the slits. Sprinkle salt and black pepper liberally over the skin and rub in. Place the chicken on a rack in a roasting pan.

Roast the chicken for about 15 minutes, then turn the oven temperature down to 350°F and bake for about 20 minutes more per pound, or until the inner thigh reaches 165°F on a meat thermometer.

NOTES

The pan drippings and carcass can be used to make roasted chicken bone broth (see page 78).

NUTRITIONAL DATA

319 calories, 21g fat, 102mg sodium, 0g fiber, 1g carbohydrates, 27g protein

1g net carbs, 3% carbs, 69% protein, 29% fat

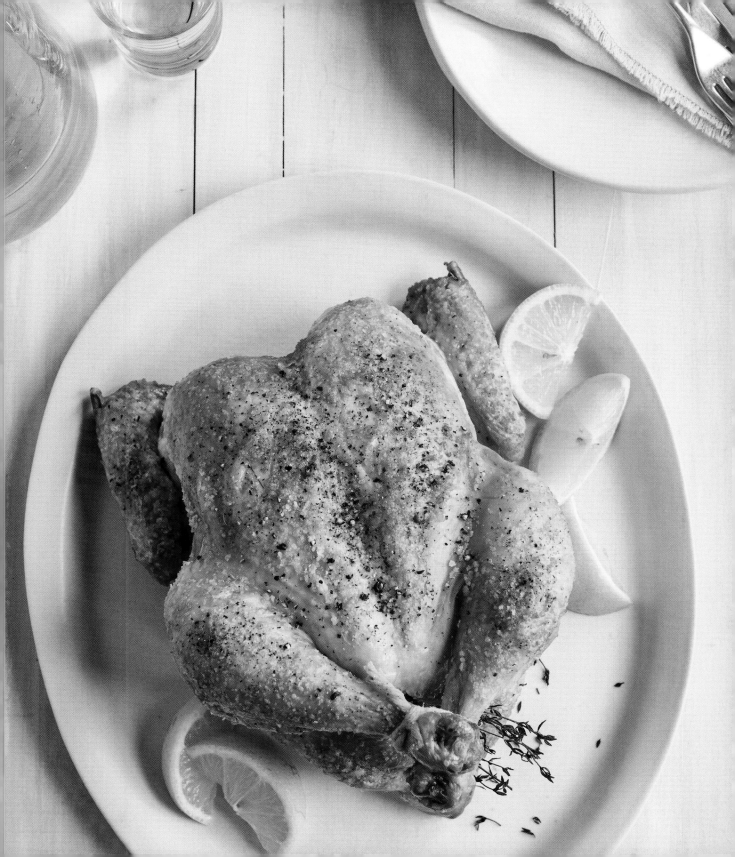

GARLIC-LEMON CHICKEN

DAIRY-FREE | NUT-FREE | EGG-FREE | PALEO, AIP

PREP TIME: 10 minutes
COOK TIME: 25 minutes
MARINATE: 3 hours
TOTAL TIME: 3 hours, 35 minutes
SERVINGS: 4

Simple yet absolutely satisfying. A simple marinade made with lemon and garlic tenderizes the meat and makes it much tastier.

¼ cup lemon juice (from about 2 lemons)

¼ cup extra-virgin olive oil

3 cloves garlic, minced

Salt and black pepper (omit pepper for AIP)

4 boneless, skinless chicken thighs

In a medium bowl, combine the lemon juice, olive oil, and garlic. Season with salt and black pepper to taste.

Add the chicken to the bowl and coat well with the marinade. Place the bowl in the refrigerator for at least 3 hours to marinate the chicken.

Preheat the oven to 400°F.

Remove the chicken from the marinade and arrange it on a shallow rimmed sheet pan. Season the chicken with additional salt and black pepper. Bake the chicken for 20 to 25 minutes, or until it reads 160°F on a meat thermometer.

NOTES

Chicken breast can be used as well, but the thighs have more fat and don't dry out as easily when cooked.

NUTRITIONAL DATA

260 calories, 18g fat, 174mg sodium, 0g fiber, 1g carbohydrates, 21g protein

1g net carbs, 2% carbs, 34% protein, 65% fat

CHICKEN-BROCCOLI CASSEROLE

NUT-FREE | EGG-FREE

PREP TIME: 10 minutes
COOK TIME: 35 minutes
TOTAL TIME: 45 minutes
SERVINGS: 8

Your family won't be complaining about having to eat yet another casserole dish when they sample this entrée. The idea is that the casserole will last all week, but don't be surprised if it's finished off in just a couple days.

1 pound broccoli florets

4 cooked chicken breasts, cubed (about 4 cups)

8 ounces cream cheese

⅓ cup heavy cream

½ teaspoon salt

2 cups shredded cheddar cheese

Preheat the oven to 350°F.

Steam the broccoli to crisp-tender, 4 to 5 minutes.

Combine the cream cheese, heavy cream, salt, and ⅓ cup water in a saucepan or microwave-safe bowl and melt over medium heat, stirring, or microwave.

In a large bowl, mix the cooked broccoli and the chicken with the sauce. Pour the mixture into a 9 × 13-inch casserole dish and top with the cheese. Bake for about 30 minutes.

NOTES

This recipe can be halved and baked in an 8 × 8-inch casserole or 2-quart round baking dish. You can also prepare it ahead, refrigerate, and bake just before serving.

NUTRITIONAL DATA

406 calories, 26g fat, 497mg sodium, 1g fiber, 5g carbohydrates, 37g protein

4g net carbs, 4% carbs, 37% protein, 59% fat

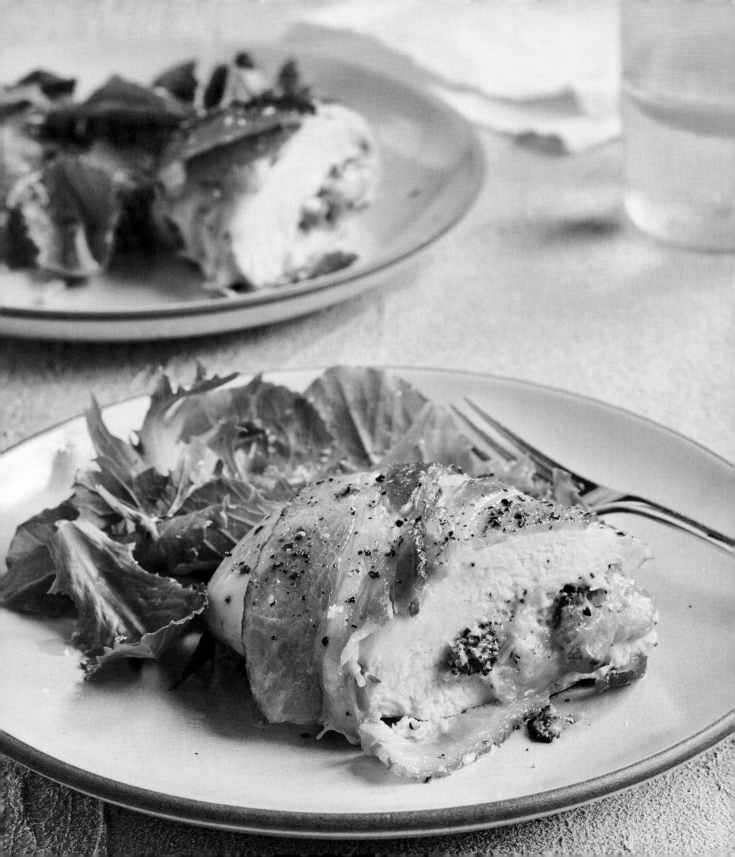

BROCCOLI AND CHEESE STUFFED CHICKEN

PREP TIME: 10 minutes
COOK TIME: 40 minutes
TOTAL TIME: 50 minutes
SERVINGS: 8

NUT-FREE

Bacon goes great with anything. Wrapping it around chicken breasts stuffed with broccoli and cheddar not only holds the stuffing in, it adds flavor and keeps the meat juicy. The dish looks gourmet, but it's so easy to prepare.

4 boneless, skinless chicken breasts

¼ teaspoon salt

Black pepper

1 cup finely chopped broccoli

1 cup shredded cheddar cheese

1 tablespoon mayonnaise

12 slices bacon

Preheat the oven to 350°F.

Season the chicken with ⅛ teaspoon of the salt and a dash of black pepper. Set aside.

In a medium bowl, combine the broccoli, cheese, mayonnaise, remaining ⅛ teaspoon salt, and a dash of black pepper. Cut a pocket into each chicken breast and stuff the broccoli mixture inside.

Wrap three pieces of bacon around each chicken breast so it covers the chicken and holds the stuffing in. Secure with toothpicks if needed.

Place the wrapped stuffed chicken breasts into a 9 × 13-inch casserole dish and bake for about 40 minutes. Remove from the oven and switch the oven to broil.

Flip each chicken piece and place under the broiler to crisp up the bacon on both sides, about 1 to 2 minutes.

NOTES

Each serving is half of a stuffed chicken breast.

> **NUTRITIONAL DATA**
>
> **314 calories, 24g fat, 485mg sodium, 0g fiber, 1g carbohydrates, 21g protein**
>
> **1g net carbs, 1% carbs, 28% protein, 71% fat**

BAKED CHICKEN THIGHS

PREP TIME: 5 minutes
COOK TIME: 35 minutes
TOTAL TIME: 40 minutes
SERVINGS: 6

DAIRY-FREE | EGG-FREE | PALEO

Ditch the high-carb bread crumbs and use seasoned almond flour instead for shake-and-bake chicken. It's a gluten-free coating the whole family will love.

1½ tablespoons extra-virgin olive oil

¼ cup almond flour

2 teaspoons salt

1 teaspoon garlic powder

1 teaspoon Italian seasoning

6 bone-in, skin-on chicken thighs

Preheat the oven to 375°F. Cover a rimmed sheet pan with aluminum foil or a silicone baking mat and drizzle the olive oil on top.

Combine the almond flour, salt, garlic powder, and Italian seasoning in a large zip-top plastic bag or mixing bowl. Shake or stir to combine. Place each piece of chicken in the bag or bowl. Shake or press to coat each piece, then place each piece on the prepared sheet pan.

Bake for 30 to 35 minutes, until the juices run clear and the coating is browned.

NOTES

A meat thermometer can be used to test doneness. Chicken thighs are fully cooked at 165°F.

Crushed pork rinds are a great alternative to almond flour for a nut-free version.

NUTRITIONAL DATA

161 calories, 8g fat, 859mg sodium, 0g fiber, 1g carbohydrates, 19g protein

1g net carbs, 3% carbs, 50% protein, 47% fat

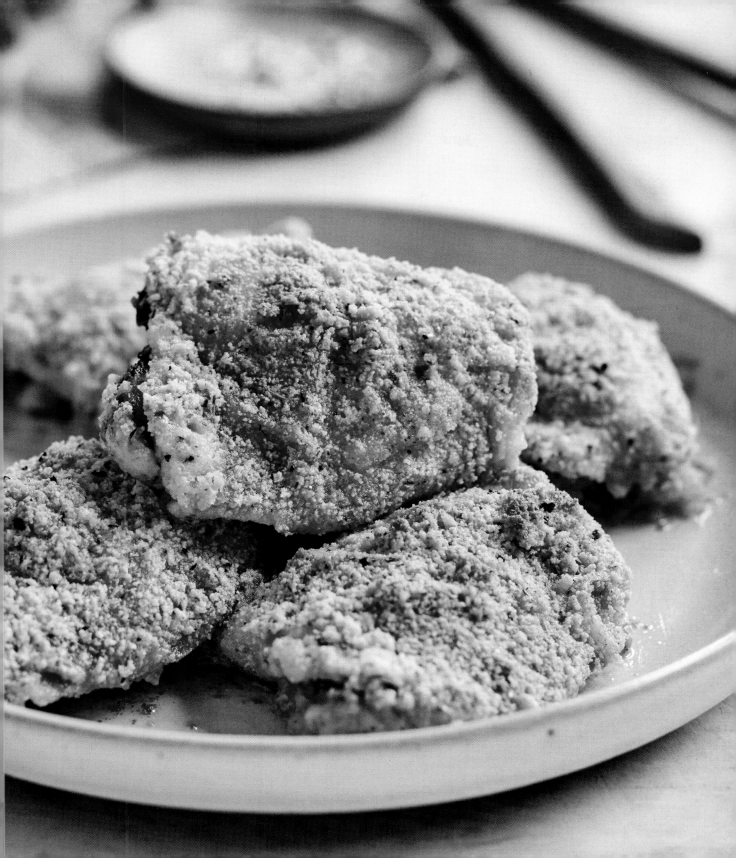

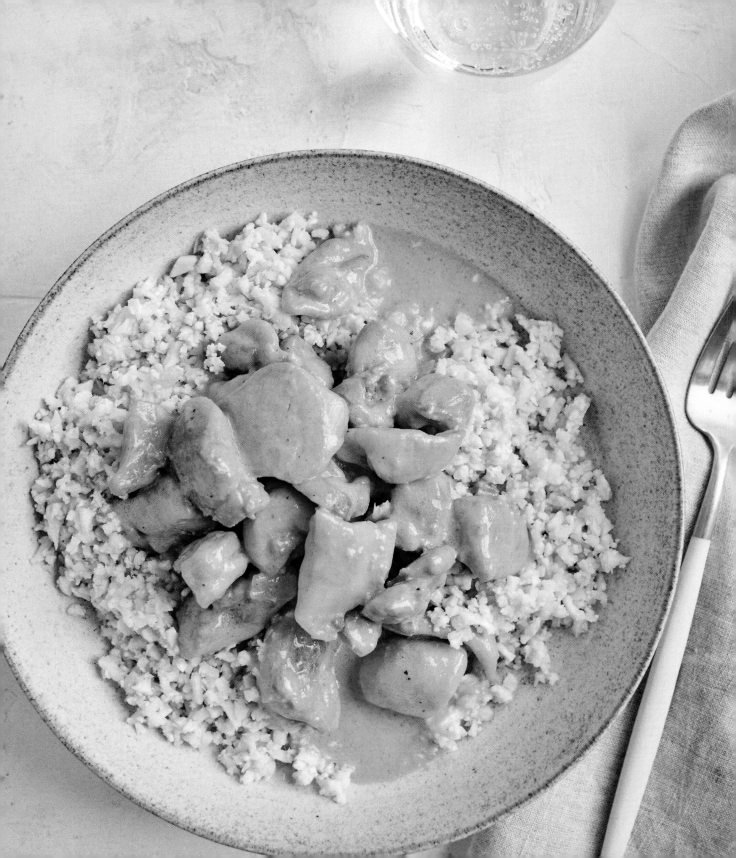

CURRIED CHICKEN

NUT-FREE | EGG-FREE

PREP TIME: 10 minutes
COOK TIME: 20 minutes
TOTAL TIME: 30 minutes
SERVINGS: 4

East meets low-carb West with this Indian-inspired dish. It's perfect for topping plain cauliflower rice.

1 tablespoon extra-virgin olive oil

1 pound boneless, skinless chicken thighs (about 4), cut into 1-inch cubes

¼ cup chopped onion

1½ teaspoons curry powder

½ teaspoon salt

¼ teaspoon ground cumin

½ cup sour cream

NOTES

Almond milk cream cheese spread or coconut cream are great dairy-free alternatives to the sour cream.

NUTRITIONAL DATA

341 calories, 28g fat, 403mg sodium, 0g fiber, 2g carbohydrates, 19g protein

2g net carbs, 2% carbs, 23% protein, 75% fat

In a medium skillet over medium-high heat, heat the oil until hot. Add the chicken and cook, stirring occasionally, until browned, 7 to 9 minutes. Stir in ⅓ cup water and the onion, curry powder, salt, and cumin. Reduce the heat, cover, and simmer until the chicken is fully cooked, about 10 minutes.

Remove from the heat and stir in the sour cream.

MARINATED TURKEY TENDERLOINS

PREP TIME: 5 minutes
COOK TIME: 40 minutes
MARINATE: 30 minutes
TOTAL TIME: 1 hour, 15 minutes
SERVINGS: 6

DAIRY-FREE | NUT-FREE | EGG-FREE | PALEO

There are so many things you can do with these marinated tenderloins. My two favorites are serving them on top of a mixed green salad or with a side of healthy, low-starch vegetables.

¼ cup coconut aminos

2 tablespoons extra-virgin olive oil

1 tablespoon Dijon mustard

2 teaspoons poultry seasoning

1½ pounds turkey tenderloins

Combine the coconut aminos, olive oil, mustard, and poultry seasoning in a gallon-size zip-top plastic bag or container. Add the turkey and marinate in the refrigerator for at least 30 minutes (preferably more than 4 hours).

Preheat the oven to 400°F.

Place the tenderloins on a sheet pan. Discard the leftover marinade. Bake for about 30 minutes, until the meat is fully cooked or reaches 165°F in the middle on a meat thermometer.

NOTES

The marinated tenderloins can also be cooked on the grill.

NUTRITIONAL DATA

172 calories, 6g fat, 644mg sodium, 0g fiber, 1g carbohydrates, 27g protein

1g net carbs, 2% carbs, 65% protein, 33% fat

SMOTHERED PORK CHOPS

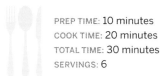

PREP TIME: 10 minutes
COOK TIME: 20 minutes
TOTAL TIME: 30 minutes
SERVINGS: 6

NUT-FREE | EGG-FREE

When you have thick pork loin chops, the best thing to do is season them first with salt and black pepper. Braising the pork in beef broth and coconut oil replaces the traditional method of caramelization, which means more healthy, satisfying fat and way less sugar and carbs.

6 boneless pork chops

1¼ teaspoons salt

Black pepper

2 tablespoons extra-virgin olive oil

1 cup beef broth

3 tablespoons coconut flour (see Note)

2 tablespoons butter

Season the pork chops with 1 teaspoon of the salt and black pepper. Heat the olive oil in a skillet over medium-high heat. Add the pork chops and brown on each side for about 5 minutes. Remove the pork chops to a plate.

In a medium bowl, combine the broth, coconut flour, and remaining ¼ teaspoon salt. Pour the broth mixture into the skillet and cook on medium heat, stirring, for about 5 minutes, until the liquid has thickened.

Return the pork chops to the skillet, cover, and cook over low heat until the pork is fully cooked, about 5 minutes. Stir in the butter to flavor and thicken the sauce. Add additional broth if it's too thick.

NOTES

The absorbency of coconut flour tends to vary, so the amount of liquid will need to be adjusted accordingly. If needed, ½ to 1 teaspoon xanthan gum or glucomannan powder can be used instead of the coconut flour for a smoother sauce.

NUTRITIONAL DATA

300 calories, 18g fat, 739mg sodium, 1g fiber, 2g carbohydrates, 30g protein

1g net carbs, 1% carbs, 34% protein, 65% fat

FILIPINO CHICKEN ADOBO

PREP TIME: 5 minutes
COOK TIME: 25 minutes
TOTAL TIME: 30 minutes
SERVINGS: 6

DAIRY-FREE | NUT-FREE | EGG-FREE | PALEO, AIP

This recipe pays homage to my Filipino heritage but with a twist. Although the flavor is similar, the cooking method is different than the traditional method. Cooking off the liquid and browning the meat makes it more flavorful. Top plain cauliflower rice with the tangy chicken for a fantastic Asian-inspired meal!

3 tablespoons apple cider vinegar

2 tablespoons extra-virgin olive oil

2 tablespoons coconut aminos

1½ teaspoons minced garlic

1½ pounds boneless chicken thighs, cut into 1- to 2-inch cubes

Mix the vinegar, oil, coconut aminos, and garlic in a cold skillet. Add the chicken and stir to coat with the vinegar mixture. The mixture can be allowed to sit for about 30 minutes, if desired, to marinate the meat.

Bring to a simmer over medium-high heat, cover, reduce the heat to medium, and simmer until the chicken is no longer pink, 10 to 12 minutes. Uncover and cook over medium-high heat, stirring occasionally, until most of the liquid has boiled off, 5 to 8 minutes. Continue cooking, flipping the chicken as needed, until the chicken is golden brown, another 3 to 5 minutes.

NOTES

It's best to use a nonstick pan for this dish to brown the outside of the meat without sticking.

To prevent overcooking the chicken while boiling off the liquid, it can be removed to a plate. Return it to the pan to brown after the liquid has reduced to only a small amount.

NUTRITIONAL DATA

295 calories, 23g fat, 423mg sodium, 0g fiber, 0g carbohydrates, 19g protein

0g net carbs, 0% carbs, 27% protein, 73% fat

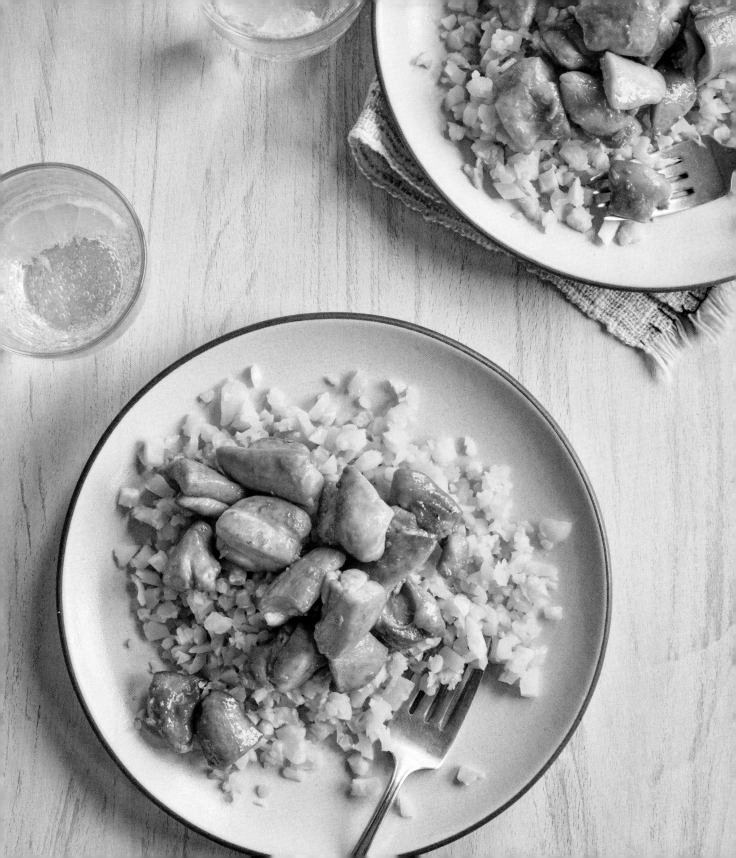

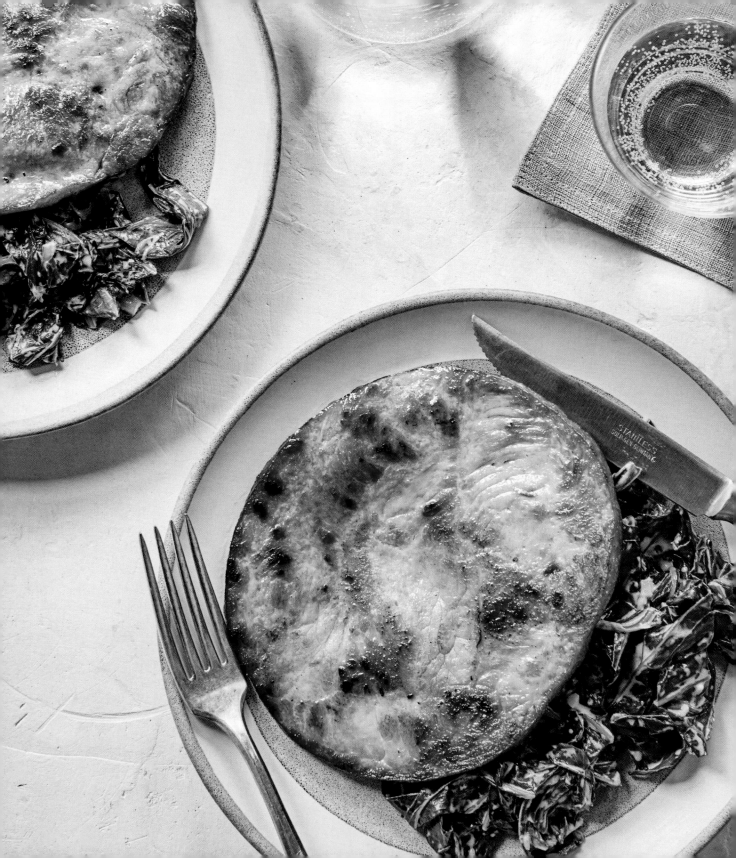

HAM AND
COLLARD GREENS

NUT-FREE | EGG-FREE

PREP TIME: 5 minutes
COOK TIME: 10 minutes
TOTAL TIME: 15 minutes
SERVINGS: 5

This classic combination is perfect for showing off your Southern hospitality!

16 ounces frozen collard greens, thawed

3 tablespoon extra-virgin olive oil

2 pounds smoked ham, cut into 5 slices

½ cup heavy cream

2 garlic cloves, minced

Drain the thawed collard greens using a wire mesh strainer to remove as much liquid as possible.

Heat the oil in a medium skillet over medium-high heat. Add the ham slices and brown on both sides, 3 to 4 minutes per side. Transfer to a plate and keep warm.

Add the collard greens, heavy cream, and garlic to the pan. Cook, stirring occasionally, until most of the liquid is absorbed, 3 to 5 minutes. Divide the greens among five plates and top each with a slice of ham.

NOTES

Kale or spinach can be used in place of the collard greens, and fresh can be used instead of frozen.

NUTRITIONAL DATA

342 calories, 24g fat, 403mg sodium, 3g fiber, 6g carbohydrates, 33g protein

3g net carbs, 3% carbs, 37% protein, 60% fat

EGG ROLL IN A BOWL

PREP TIME: 5 minutes
COOK TIME: 15 minutes
TOTAL TIME: 20 minutes
SERVINGS: 6

DAIRY-FREE | NUT-FREE | EGG-FREE | PALEO, AIP

Have egg rolls but hold the rolls! The egg roll filling is the best part anyway, so why bother with the carb-y wrapper? If you need a blanket for the filling, wrap it in lettuce.

1 pound ground pork

1 (16-ounce) bag coleslaw mix

¼ cup coconut aminos

3 cloves garlic

½ teaspoon ground ginger

In a large skillet over medium heat, cook the ground pork, stirring and breaking it up with a wooden spoon, until no longer pink, 7 to 10 minutes. Add the coleslaw mix, coconut aminos, garlic, and ginger and cook, stirring, until the cabbage is wilted, 3 to 5 minutes.

NOTES

A sprinkling of Chinese five-spice powder can be added for more zing, and green onions can be added for garnish.

NUTRITIONAL DATA

225 calories, 16g fat, 596mg sodium, 1g fiber, 5g carbohydrates, 14g protein

4g net carbs, 7% carbs, 26% protein, 67% fat

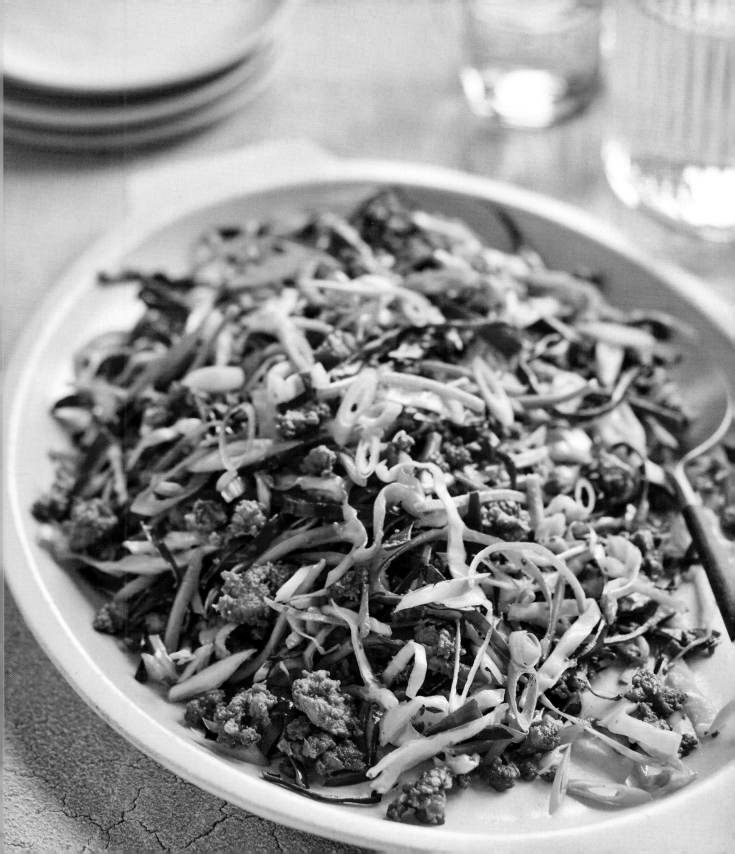

PORK LOIN ROAST

DAIRY-FREE | NUT-FREE | EGG-FREE | PALEO, AIP

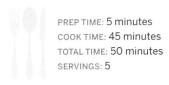

PREP TIME: 5 minutes
COOK TIME: 45 minutes
TOTAL TIME: 50 minutes
SERVINGS: 5

After you quickly season the pork loin, you'll have plenty of time on your hands while it's cooking. Go ahead and watch a couple episodes of your favorite show. Serve it with Almond Asparagus (page 111) for a memorable meal.

1 teaspoon garlic salt

1 teaspoon dried thyme

1 teaspoon ground cumin (omit for AIP)

1 teaspoon dried oregano

¼ teaspoon black pepper (omit for AIP)

1½ pounds boneless pork loin roast

Preheat the oven to 350°F. Lightly grease a medium sheet pan.

Mix the garlic salt, thyme, cumin, oregano, and black pepper together in a small bowl. Rub the garlic salt mixture evenly onto the pork roast. Transfer to the prepared sheet pan.

Bake the pork roast for about 45 minutes or to an internal temperature of 145° to 160°F. Allow to rest for at least 10 minutes before slicing.

NUTRITIONAL DATA

184 calories, 5g fat, 300mg sodium, 0g fiber, 1g carbohydrates, 30g protein

1g net carbs, 2% carbs, 71% protein, 27% fat

CHICKEN WITH SPINACH AND TOMATO

PREP TIME: 10 minutes
COOK TIME: 20 minutes
TOTAL TIME: 30 minutes
SERVINGS: 6

DAIRY-FREE | NUT-FREE | EGG-FREE | PALEO

A classic high-protein, nutrient-dense meal for the whole family that cooks up in one pot. And if there are leftovers, you can enjoy it for lunch the next day too.

3 tablespoons extra-virgin olive oil

2 pounds boneless, skinless chicken thighs, diced into 1-inch pieces

2 cloves garlic, minced

½ teaspoon salt (¼ teaspoon if using salted canned tomatoes)

⅛ teaspoon black pepper

1 (15-ounce) can diced tomatoes, undrained

8 ounces mushrooms, thinly sliced

7½ cups (5 ounces) baby spinach

NOTES

Each serving can be sprinkled with Parmesan cheese.

NUTRITIONAL DATA

269 calories, 13g fat, 451mg sodium, 1g fiber, 5g carbohydrates, 31g protein

4g net carbs, 6% carbs, 48% protein, 46% fat

Add the olive oil to large pot and place over medium heat. When the oil is hot, add the chicken and garlic and season with the salt and black pepper. Cook, stirring, until the chicken is no longer pink, 5 to 7 minutes.

Add the tomatoes, mushrooms, and spinach and cook, stirring occasionally, until the liquid is reduced by about half, 12 to 15 minutes. Adjust the seasonings if needed.

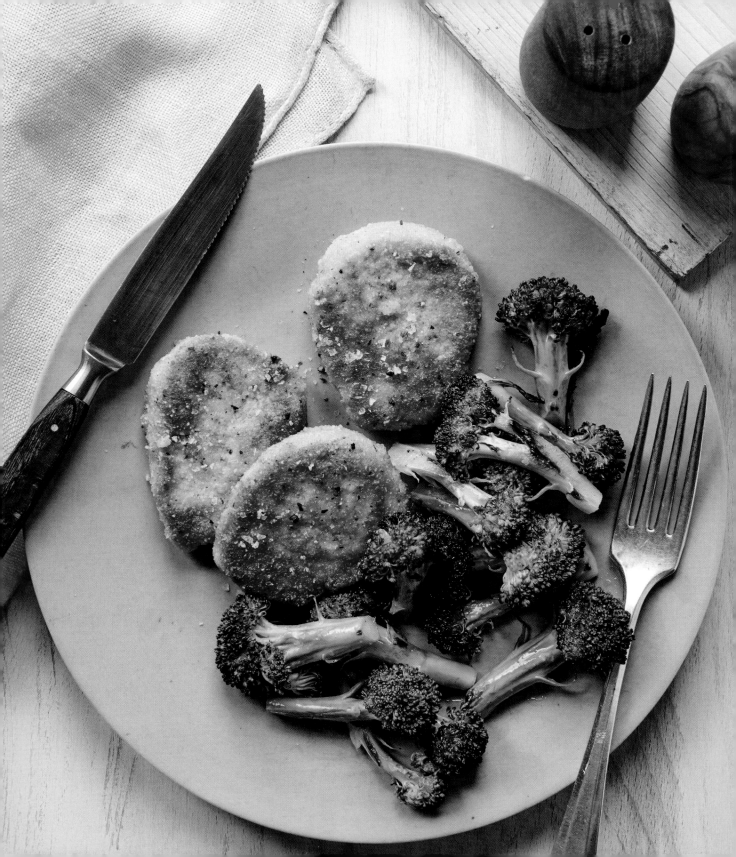

QUICK "BREADED" PORK

PREP TIME: 15 minutes
COOK TIME: 10 minutes
TOTAL TIME: 20 minutes
SERVINGS: 4

DAIRY-FREE | PALEO

A Southern classic with pork tenderloin medallions made low-carb and keto friendly. But I bet even in the heart of Dixie no one would miss the unnecessary carbs!

½ cup finely ground almond flour

3 tablespoons coconut flour

½ teaspoon Italian seasoning

½ teaspoon salt

¼ teaspoon black pepper

1 pound pork tenderloin

1 large egg

3 tablespoons avocado oil

In a large zip-top plastic bag, combine the almond flour, coconut flour, Italian seasoning, salt, and black pepper. Set aside.

Put the egg in a shallow bowl and lightly beat. Cut the tenderloin into ½-inch-thick slices. Dip each cutlet in the egg, then shake in the bag with the coconut flour mixture to coat.

Heat the oil in a large skillet over medium-high heat. Add the tenderloin cutlets and cook until browned, 2 to 4 minutes per side.

NOTES

Use tongs to gently turn each piece to brown both sides without losing the coating.

Serve with Parmesan cheese sprinkled on top, if desired.

NUTRITIONAL DATA

346 calories, 23g fat, 376mg sodium, 3g fiber, 6g carbohydrates, 28g protein

3g net carbs, 4% carbs, 34% protein, 63% fat

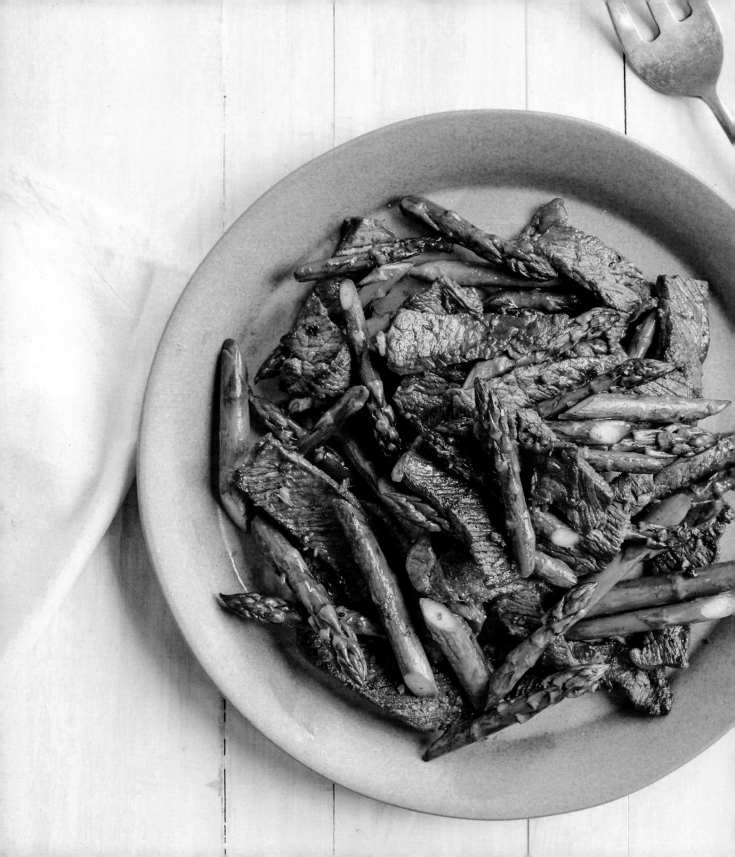

MAIN DISHES: BEEF AND LAMB

Rib-Eye Steaks in Red Wine Sauce 142

Beef Filet with Mushrooms 144

Zucchini Meatloaf 145

Lamb Patties 147

Ginger Beef and Asparagus 148

Ground Beef and Cabbage 150

Pepper Steak 151

Beef Pot Roast 153

No-Noodle Lasagna 154

Stuffed Peppers 156

Cheeseburger Casserole 157

Steak Pinwheels 159

Garlic Lamb Chops 160

Braised Short Ribs 163

RIB-EYE STEAKS IN RED WINE SAUCE

PREP TIME: 10 minutes
COOK TIME: 15 minutes
TOTAL TIME: 25 minutes
SERVINGS: 4

NUT-FREE | EGG-FREE

Did you know that combining a little red wine and butter makes for an incredibly tasty and hassle-free homemade steak sauce? I wouldn't pop open your most expensive bottle of Château Margaux—any decent red will make the steak pop with flavor.

1½ pounds boneless rib-eye steaks

¼ teaspoon salt

Dash black pepper

1 tablespoon extra-virgin olive oil

2 cloves garlic, minced

⅓ cup dry red wine

2 tablespoons butter

1 tablespoon chopped fresh parsley (optional), for garnish

NOTES

Butter-flavored coconut oil can be used in place of butter to make this dairy-free.

NUTRITIONAL DATA

454 calories, 33g fat, 211mg sodium, 0g fiber, 1g carbohydrates, 34g protein

1g net carbs, 1% carbs, 31% protein, 68% fat

Season both sides of the steaks with salt and black pepper.

Heat the oil in a large skillet over medium-high heat. Add the garlic and cook, stirring, until fragrant, about a minute. Add the steaks and cook for 3 to 5 minutes on each side, or to desired doneness. Remove the steaks from the pan and keep warm.

Pour in the wine and boil until reduced to about 2 tablespoons, about 2 minutes. Remove from the heat and stir in the butter. Spoon the sauce over the steaks.

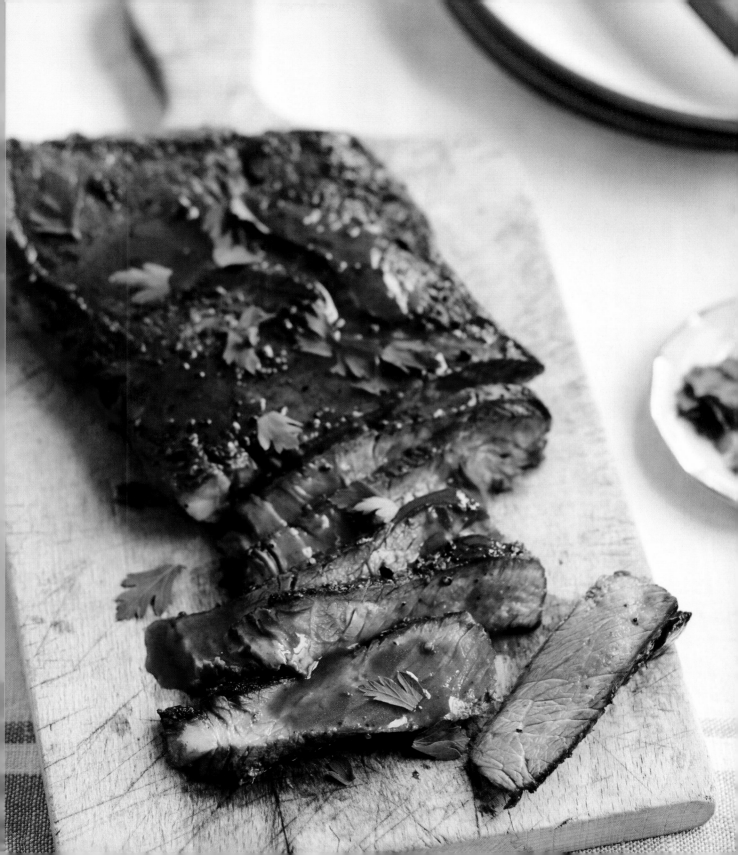

BEEF FILET WITH MUSHROOMS

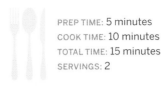

PREP TIME: 5 minutes
COOK TIME: 10 minutes
TOTAL TIME: 15 minutes
SERVINGS: 2

DAIRY-FREE | NUT-FREE | EGG-FREE | PALEO, AIP

Steak and mushrooms . . . such a classic combination. Using the highly prized tender filet mignon cut provides a rich meal that takes little time to prepare.

2 beef filet mignon steaks (about 12 ounces total)

⅛ teaspoon salt

Dash black pepper (omit for AIP)

3 tablespoons extra-virgin olive oil

1 cup sliced mushrooms (see Notes)

1 teaspoon dried thyme

½ cup chopped green onions (optional), for garnish

Season the meat with the salt and black pepper

Heat 1 tablespoon of the olive oil in a large skillet over medium heat. Add the steaks and cook for 2 to 3 minutes per side, or to desired doneness. Remove from the pan and keep warm.

Add the remaining 2 tablespoons oil to the pan along with the mushrooms and thyme and cook, stirring, until the mushrooms are softened, about 2 minutes.

Serve the steaks with the mushrooms spooned over the top. Garnish with the green onions if desired.

NOTES

Any mushroom can be used, but shiitakes and portobellas are favorites of mine.

NUTRITIONAL DATA

609 calories, 51g fat, 235g sodium, 1g fiber, 3g carbohydrates, 32g protein

2g net carbs, 1% carbs, 22% protein, 77% fat

ZUCCHINI MEATLOAF

DAIRY-FREE | NUT-FREE | PALEO

PREP TIME: 10 minutes
COOK TIME: 1 hour
TOTAL TIME: 1 hour, 10 minutes
SERVINGS: 8

Adding shredded zucchini into meatloaf is a sneaky way to get kids to eat their veggies, as well as a way to keep the meat moist while baking.

Coconut oil (optional), for greasing

2 pounds ground beef

1 medium zucchini, shredded (1½ packed cups)

2 large eggs, lightly beaten

⅓ cup tomato sauce

2 tablespoons coconut flour

2 tablespoons dried parsley (optional)

½ teaspoon salt

⅛ teaspoon black pepper

Preheat the oven to 350°F. Grease a rimmed baking sheet with coconut oil or line with a silicone baking mat or parchment paper.

In a bowl, mix together the ground beef, zucchini, eggs, tomato sauce, coconut flour, parsley (if using), salt, and black pepper. Shape into a loaf on the prepared sheet pan.

Bake for about 1 hour. Remove any liquid collected at the bottom of the pan. Allow the meatloaf to rest for at least 5 minutes before slicing.

NOTES

Add about ½ cup chopped onions if you don't mind the extra carbs. Or change it up using half ground beef and half sausage meat.

Spreading a layer of Low-Carb Ketchup (page 95) over the top of the meatloaf at the end of baking adds a touch of sweetness.

NUTRITIONAL DATA

318 calories, 24g fat, 296mg sodium, 1g fiber, 2g carbohydrates, 22g protein

1g net carbs, 1% carbs, 29% protein, 70% fat

VARIATIONS

Mexican: Add 1 (4-ounce) can drained chopped chiles, 3 minced cloves garlic, 1½ teaspoons ground cumin, and ¼ teaspoon red pepper flakes. Serve with grated cheese and sour cream.

Italian: Add ¾ cup mozzarella cheese, 3 minced cloves garlic, 1 teaspoon dried basil, and 1 teaspoon dried oregano.

Greek: Add 10 ounces frozen chopped spinach (thawed and drained), 3 minced cloves garlic, ⅓ cup pitted and chopped Kalamata olives, and ½ cup feta cheese, if desired.

Bacon Cheeseburger: Add 1 cup grated cheddar cheese and place uncooked slices of bacon over the loaf before baking.

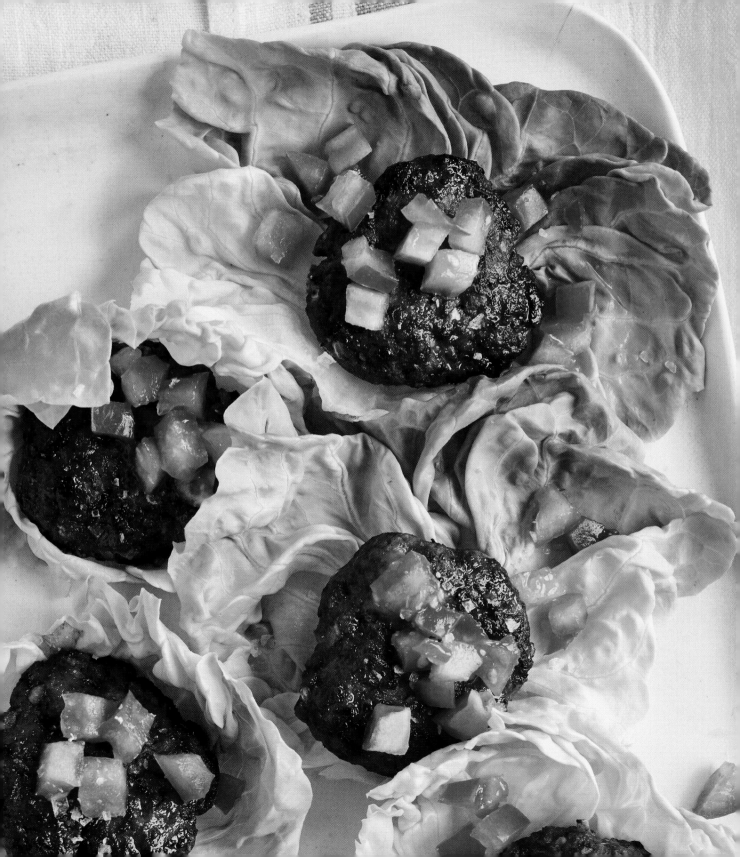

LAMB PATTIES

DAIRY-FREE | NUT-FREE | EGG-FREE | PALEO

PREP TIME: 10 minutes
COOK TIME: 10 minutes
TOTAL TIME: 20 minutes
SERVINGS: 6

Mix up the red meat from time to time with lamb. Ounce for ounce, it's got more iron than beef, and I think seasoned ground lamb meat makes for a more satisfying burger. Just don't drown it in ketchup! Serve them plain, in a lettuce wrap, or between two slices of Almond Flour Bread (page 70).

1½ pounds ground lamb

¼ cup finely chopped onion

2 cloves garlic, finely chopped

1 teaspoon ground cumin

1 teaspoon salt

½ teaspoon ground coriander

½ teaspoon black pepper

Combine the lamb, onion, garlic, cumin, salt, coriander, and black pepper in a large bowl and mix with your hands to blend well. Shape into 6 patties about ½ inch thick.

Cook the patties in a large skillet over medium-high heat, turning once, until the meat is browned outside and no longer pink inside, about 10 minutes. (They're also great if you grill them.)

NUTRITIONAL DATA

325 calories, 26g fat, 455mg sodium, 0g fiber, 1g carbohydrates, 18g protein

1g net carbs, 1% carbs, 23% protein, 75% fat

GINGER BEEF AND ASPARAGUS

PREP TIME: 7 minutes
COOK TIME: 8 minutes
TOTAL TIME: 15 minutes
SERVINGS: 5

DAIRY-FREE | NUT-FREE | EGG-FREE | PALEO, AIP

Take a virtual culinary trip around the world with this Asian-inspired vegetable stir-fry. The seasonings will remind you of your favorite Thai restaurant, but you'll save money on the bill.

1¼ pounds sirloin beef

¼ teaspoon salt

¼ teaspoon black pepper (omit for AIP)

3 tablespoons avocado oil

¾ pound thin asparagus spears, cut into 2-inch pieces

1 tablespoon finely chopped fresh ginger

2 cloves garlic, finely chopped

2 tablespoons coconut aminos

Cut the beef against the grain into thin strips and season with the salt and black pepper.

In a large skillet, heat the oil over high heat. Add the beef and cook, stirring, until it's no longer pink, about 2 minutes. Add the asparagus and cook, stirring, for 1 to 2 minutes. Add the ginger and garlic and cook, stirring, until fragrant, about 1 minute.

Reduce the heat to medium. Add the coconut aminos and stir it in. Cook, stirring, for another 1 to 2 minutes.

NOTES

Green beans can be subbed for the asparagus, if desired.

NUTRITIONAL DATA

231 calories, 12g fat, 268mg sodium, 1g fiber, 3g carbohydrates, 26g protein

2g net carbs, 4% carbs, 47% protein, 49% fat

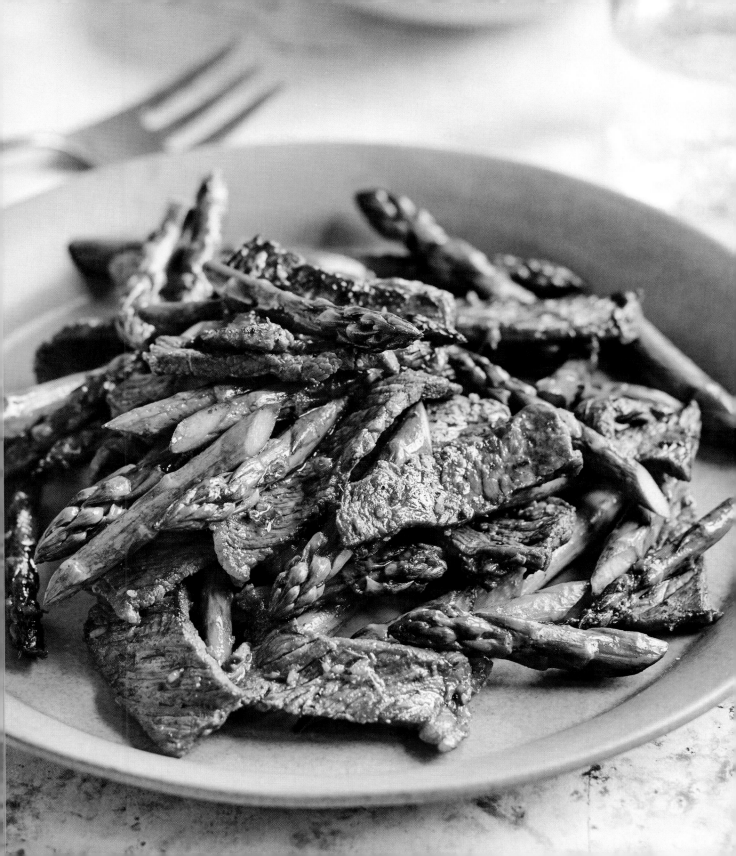

GROUND BEEF AND CABBAGE

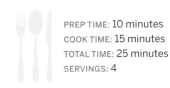

PREP TIME: 10 minutes
COOK TIME: 15 minutes
TOTAL TIME: 25 minutes
SERVINGS: 4

DAIRY-FREE | NUT-FREE | EGG-FREE | PALEO

So good, I could honestly eat this simple skillet dish every week and not get tired of it. You'll want to break out the cast-iron skillet for this one!

1 pound ground beef

¼ cup chopped onion

1 clove garlic, minced

⅛ teaspoon salt

Dash black pepper

2 cups shredded cabbage (about ⅓ small head)

½ cup tomato sauce

Heat a cast-iron skillet over medium-high heat. Add the ground beef, onions, garlic, salt, and black pepper and cook, stirring and breaking up the beef with a wooden spoon, until the beef is browned. Remove the cooked beef to a plate.

Add the cabbage to the beef fat in the skillet and cook, stirring, until wilted, 3 to 5 minutes. Stir in the tomato sauce and beef mixture and cook, stirring occasionally, for about 10 minutes.

NOTES

A whole (8-ounce) can of tomato sauce can be used, but it will add about 1.5g net carbs per serving.

NUTRITIONAL DATA

309 calories, 23g fat, 316mg sodium, 2g fiber, 5g carbohydrates, 20g protein

4g net carbs, 4% carbs, 27% protein, 69% fat

PEPPER STEAK

DAIRY-FREE | NUT-FREE | EGG-FREE | PALEO

PREP TIME: 10 minutes
COOK TIME: 20 minutes
TOTAL TIME: 30 minutes
SERVINGS: 8

Transform everyday pepper steak into a healthy dish by adding cabbage, which makes the steak more flavorful. Plus, you'll probably eat less of the meat, leaving more for leftovers.

1 pound steak

Salt and black pepper

¼ teaspoon red pepper flakes

3 tablespoons avocado oil

1 head cabbage

1 medium red bell pepper

2 tablespoons coconut aminos

Slice the steak into thin strips. Season generously with salt and black pepper, and sprinkle on the red pepper flakes.

Heat 2 tablespoons of the oil in a large skillet or wok. Add the meat and cook, turning occasionally, until browned, 5 to 7 minutes.

While the meat is browning, prepare the vegetables. Roughly chop the cabbage. Slice the bell pepper into bite-size strips.

After the meat is browned, add the cabbage and bell pepper. Reduce the heat to maintain a simmer, cover, and cook, stirring occasionally, until the cabbage is wilted, about 10 minutes.

Sprinkle in the coconut aminos and cook, stirring, for another 1 to 2 minutes.

NOTES

To make slicing the steak easier, freeze it for 15 minutes or so before slicing.

Other vegetables like celery, mushrooms, or squash can be added.

NUTRITIONAL DATA

157 calories, 8g fat, 339mg sodium, 3g fiber, 7g carbohydrates, 13g protein

4g net carbs, 11% carbs, 37% protein, 52% fat

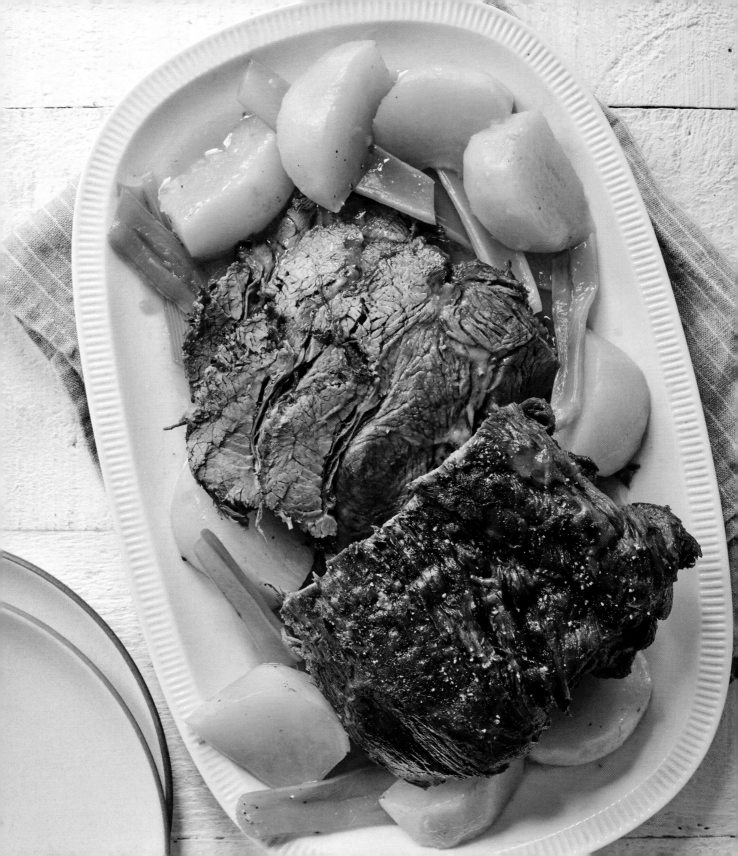

BEEF POT ROAST

DAIRY-FREE | NUT-FREE | EGG-FREE

PREP TIME: 10 minutes
COOK TIME: 2 hours, 15 minutes
TOTAL TIME: 2 hours, 25 minutes
SERVINGS: 8

Nobody's going to question where you're hiding the carrots. The beef, veggies, and sauce are so good that there's no need for high-sugar veggies.

3½ pounds beef roast

½ teaspoon salt

⅛ teaspoon black pepper

2 tablespoons extra-virgin olive oil

½ teaspoon dried basil

½ teaspoon Worcestershire sauce

2 medium turnips, peeled and quartered

4 stalks celery

Season the roast with the salt and black pepper. Heat the oil in a Dutch oven over medium-high heat. Add the roast and brown the meat slowly on all sides, about 10 minutes. Add 1 cup water, the basil, and Worcestershire sauce. Reduce heat, cover, and simmer for 1 to 1½ hours.

Add the turnips and celery. Season with more salt and black pepper, if desired. (I added about ½ teaspoon salt.) Cover and cook until the vegetables are tender, about 45 minutes.

NOTES

You can slow-cook this roast in the oven, if you prefer: After browning the meat, place the covered Dutch oven in a preheated 325°F oven and bake 1 to 1½ hours. Add the vegetables, cover, and return the pot to the oven for another 45 minutes to cook the vegetables to tender.

NUTRITIONAL DATA

397 calories, 26g fat, 186mg sodium, 0g fiber, 2g carbohydrates, 38g protein

2g net carbs, 2% carbs, 39% protein, 59% fat

NO-NOODLE LASAGNA

NUT-FREE | EGG-FREE

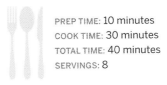

PREP TIME: 10 minutes
COOK TIME: 30 minutes
TOTAL TIME: 40 minutes
SERVINGS: 8

What's lasagna without the noodles? Scrumptious ground beef and cheese without the belly-bloating carbs.

1 pound ground beef
⅛ teaspoon salt
Dash black pepper
1½ cups ricotta cheese
½ cup grated Parmesan cheese
1 (25-ounce) jar marinara sauce
8 ounces mozzarella cheese, sliced

NOTES

An egg can be mixed into the ricotta before layering.

NUTRITIONAL DATA

355 calories, 25g fat, 838mg sodium, 1g fiber, 7g carbohydrates, 24g protein

6g net carbs, 7% carbs, 28% protein, 65% fat

Preheat the oven to 350°F. Season the ground beef with the salt and black pepper. Heat a large skillet over medium heat. Add the beef and cook, stirring and breaking up the meat with a wooden spoon, until browned. Drain off any excess fat.

Transfer the beef to the bottom of a 9 × 9-inch baking pan. Spread the ricotta on top, followed by the Parmesan. Then pour the marinara sauce over the layers and top with the mozzarella.

Bake for 25 minutes.

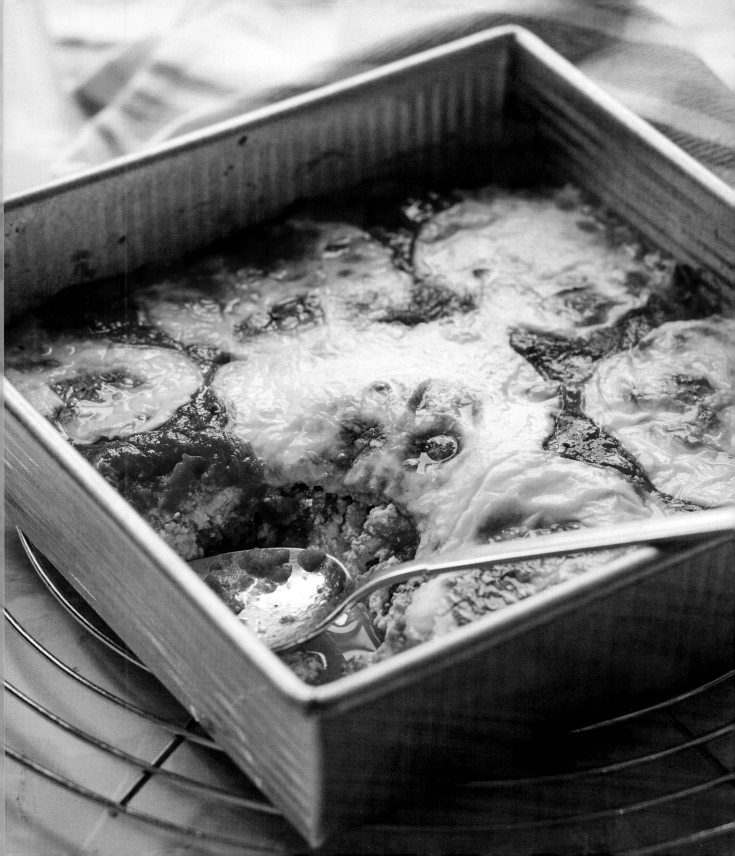

STUFFED PEPPERS

DAIRY-FREE | NUT-FREE | EGG-FREE | PALEO

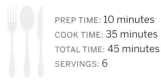

PREP TIME: 10 minutes
COOK TIME: 35 minutes
TOTAL TIME: 45 minutes
SERVINGS: 6

Instead of stuffing peppers with high-carb rice, pair the ground beef with riced cauliflower. No bowl needed—the pepper is the bowl!

1¼ pounds ground beef

¼ cup chopped onion

2 cups riced cauliflower (see page 109)

8 ounces tomato sauce

½ teaspoon salt

Dash black pepper

6 medium green bell peppers

Preheat the oven to 375°F.

Heat a large skillet over medium heat and add the beef and onion. Cook, stirring and breaking up the beef with a wooden spoon, until the beef is browned. Drain the fat from the skillet, if desired. Add the riced cauliflower and cook, stirring, for 3 to 5 minutes. Remove from the heat and stir in the tomato sauce, salt, and black pepper.

Cut the tops off the bell peppers and scoop out and remove the seeds. Stand the peppers upright in a casserole dish. Fill each pepper with the ground beef mixture.

Bake, covered, for 20 to 25 minutes, or until the peppers are tender.

NOTES

For those who can have dairy, these are great topped with a shredded cheese blend like mozzarella and Colby Jack before baking.

NUTRITIONAL DATA

283 calories, 19g fat, 469mg sodium, 3g fiber, 9g carbohydrates, 18g protein

6g net carbs, 9% carbs, 27% protein, 64% fat

CHEESEBURGER CASSEROLE

NUT-FREE

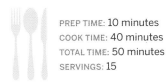

PREP TIME: 10 minutes
COOK TIME: 40 minutes
TOTAL TIME: 50 minutes
SERVINGS: 15

Why make just one burger with a high-carb bun when you can make a filling casserole that makes enough for a crowd with hardly any carbs. No buns? No problem!

2 pounds ground beef

½ teaspoon salt

¼ teaspoon black pepper

8 large eggs

1 cup heavy cream

12 ounces cheddar cheese, grated

1 teaspoon garlic salt

Preheat the oven to 350°F.

Season the ground beef with the salt and black pepper. Add the beef to a large skillet over medium-high heat and cook, stirring and breaking up the meat with a wooden spoon, until browned. Drain any excess fat if needed. Then spread the beef over the bottom of a 9 × 13-inch casserole dish.

In a bowl, whisk together the eggs, cream, three-quarters of the cheese, and the garlic salt. Pour over the beef. Top with the remaining cheese.

Bake for 30 to 35 minutes, until the top is golden.

NOTES

The measures can be cut in half and the casserole baked in an 8 × 8-inch pan for fewer servings.

For a bacon cheeseburger, add chopped cooked bacon to the beef.

For a mushroom burger, add sliced white button mushrooms to the beef.

Great served with ketchup, pickles, mustard, and other burger fixings.

NUTRITIONAL DATA

333 calories, 28g fat, 376mg sodium, 0g fiber, 1g carbohydrates, 19g protein

1g net carbs, 1% carbs, 23% protein, 75% fat

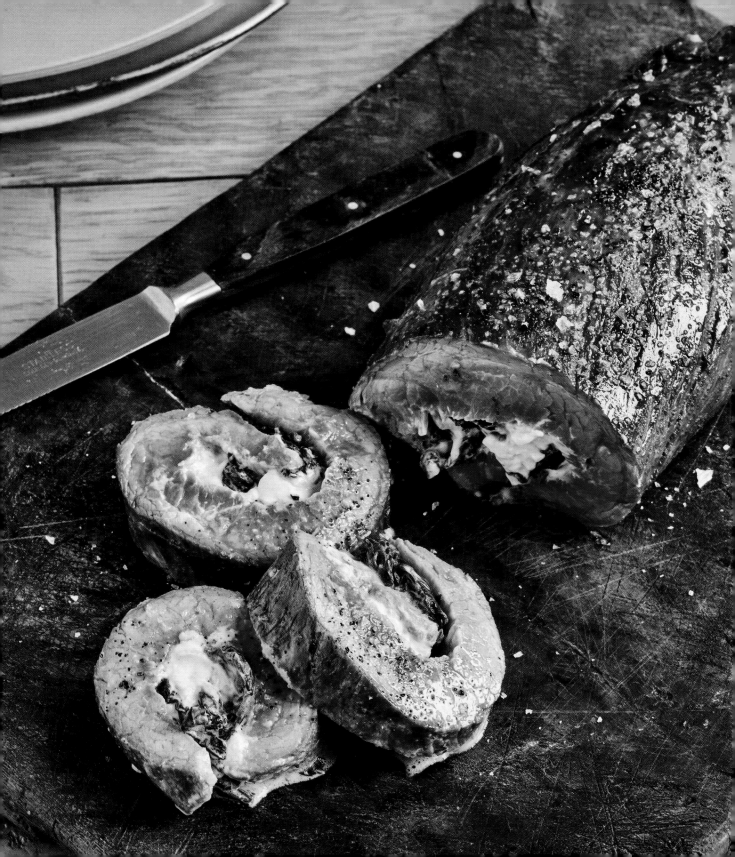

STEAK PINWHEELS

NUT-FREE | EGG-FREE

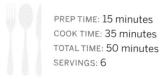

PREP TIME: 15 minutes
COOK TIME: 35 minutes
TOTAL TIME: 50 minutes
SERVINGS: 6

Is it okay to eat steak with your hands? Sure, why not? Steak pinwheels with spinach and cheese are a finger food that's sure to impress your family and guests.

1½ pounds thin flank steak

Salt and black pepper

3 tablespoons extra-virgin olive oil

7½ cups (5 ounces) baby spinach

4 ounces cream cheese, softened

2 tablespoons grated Parmesan cheese

3 cloves garlic, minced

Preheat the oven to 350°F.

Season the steak liberally with salt and black pepper. Set aside.

Heat half of the oil in a skillet over medium heat. Add the spinach and cook, stirring, until wilted, 2 to 3 minutes. Remove from the heat.

In a bowl, combine the cream cheese, Parmesan, and garlic. Spread onto one side of the steak. Top with the spinach. Roll the steak into a log and secure with toothpicks.

Drizzle a rimmed sheet pan with the remaining oil. Place the steak in the pan with the seam side up. Bake for 25 to 30 minutes, until cooked to medium doneness.

Allow the meat to rest for least 10 minutes before slicing and remove the toothpicks before serving.

NOTES

Any thin steak can be used.

NUTRITIONAL DATA

296 calories, 19g fat, 166mg sodium, 0g fiber, 2g carbohydrates, 26g protein

2g net carbs, 3% carbs, 37% protein, 60% fat

GARLIC LAMB CHOPS

DAIRY-FREE | NUT-FREE | EGG-FREE | PALEO, AIP

PREP TIME: 10 minutes
COOK TIME: 15 minutes
MARINATE: 1 hour
TOTAL TIME: 1 hour 25 minutes
SERVINGS: 4

Although lamb chops are tasty plain, a simple marinade makes them more tender and flavorful.

½ onion, sliced

3 tablespoons apple cider vinegar

3 tablespoons extra-virgin olive oil

1 tablespoon minced garlic

1 teaspoon salt

1 pound lamb chops

Combine the onion, vinegar, olive oil, garlic, and salt in a large zip-top plastic bag. Add the lamb chops and marinate in the refrigerator for an hour.

Preheat the oven to 425°F.

In an oven-safe skillet over medium-high heat, sear lamb chops for about 3 minutes per side. Transfer the skillet to the oven and bake for 6 to 8 minutes, until done (the lamb should register 140°F on a meat thermometer at its thickest point).

NUTRITIONAL DATA

293 calories, 18g fat, 649mg sodium, 0g fiber, 2g carbohydrates, 28g protein

0g net carbs, 0% carbs, 49% protein, 51% fat

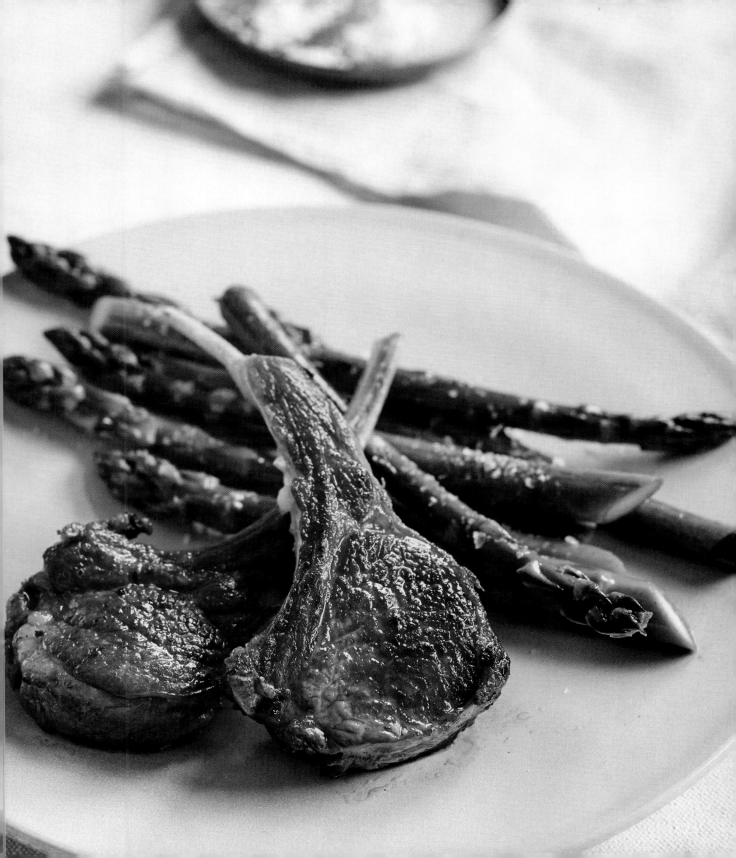

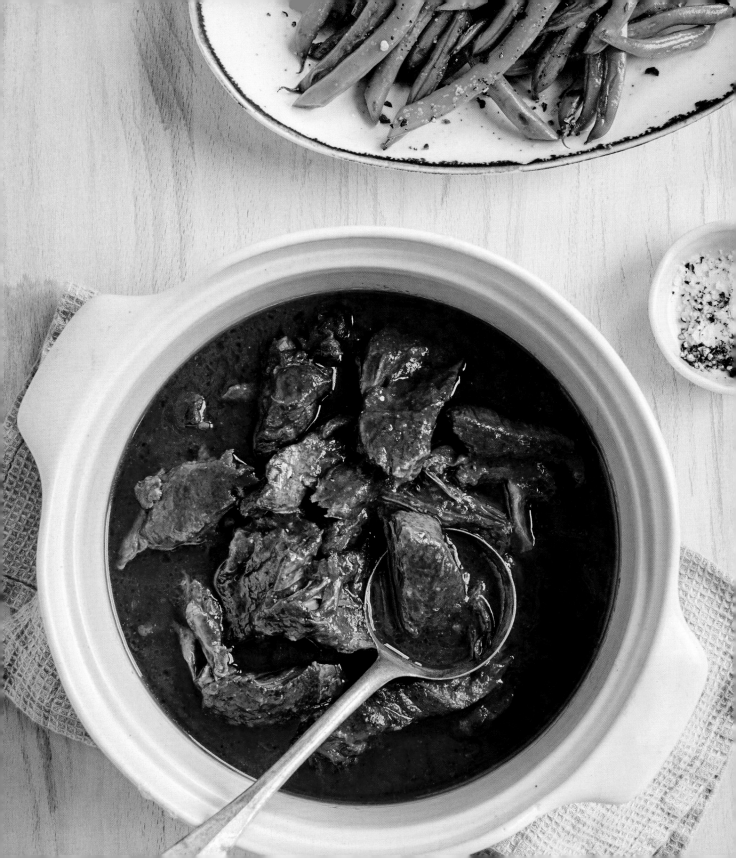

BRAISED SHORT RIBS

DAIRY-FREE | NUT-FREE | EGG-FREE | PALEO

PREP TIME: 10 minutes
COOK TIME: 2 hours, 5 minutes
TOTAL TIME: 2 hours, 15 minutes
SERVINGS: 8

The challenge with this recipe is patiently waiting while the ribs are slowly simmering. Don't jump the gun and devour them before they become super tender and loaded with flavor.

2 pounds boneless beef short ribs

Salt and black pepper

3 tablespoons extra-virgin olive oil

2 cups beef broth

¼ cup tomato paste

½ teaspoon fresh thyme

½ teaspoon garlic powder

Season the meat with salt and black pepper. Heat the oil in a Dutch oven over high heat. Add the short ribs and sear the meat on all sides, 10 to 12 minutes total.

Pour in the broth. Stir in the tomato paste, thyme, and garlic powder and sprinkle in salt and black pepper to taste. Reduce the heat to maintain a simmer, cover, and cook for 2 hours.

NOTES

A tablespoon of Worcestershire sauce can be added for extra flavor.

NUTRITIONAL DATA

254 calories, 16g fat, 434mg sodium, 0g fiber, 1g carbohydrates, 22g protein

1g net carbs, 2% carbs, 37% protein, 61% fat

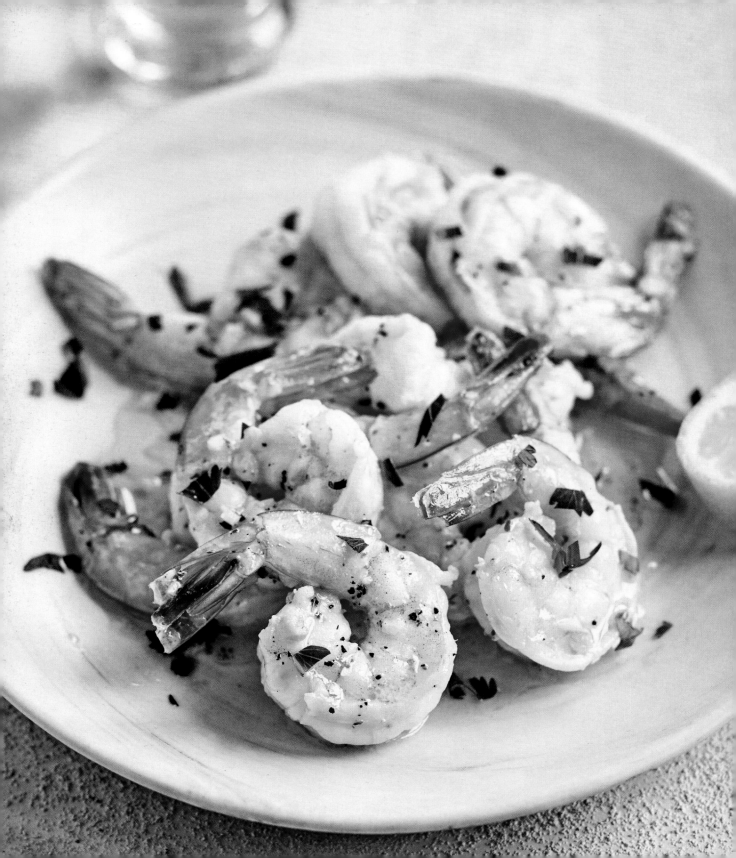

MAIN DISHES: SEAFOOD

Fish Florentine 166

Salmon with Creamy Dill Sauce 166

Crab Quiche 169

Shrimp Scampi 170

Stir-Fried Scallops 173

Garlicky Steamed Mussels 174

Baked Flounder with Tomato 177

Balsamic Halibut 178

Tuna Casserole 179

Butter Fish 180

Creamy Clam Sauce over Zoodles 181

"Breaded" Flounder 182

FISH FLORENTINE

NUT-FREE

PREP TIME: 10 minutes	**COOK TIME:** 45 minutes
TOTAL TIME: 55 minutes	**SERVINGS:** 6

Obsessed with spinach? Love fish entrées? Marry them together and top with a tangy Parmesan sauce.

¾ cup grated Parmesan

¾ cup mayonnaise

½ cup sour cream

12 ounces frozen spinach, thawed and drained, or about 1 pound fresh

1½ pounds cod fillets or similar fish

Preheat the oven to 350°F. Lightly grease a 9 × 13-inch casserole dish.

In small bowl, mix together the Parmesan cheese, mayonnaise, and sour cream.

Layer the spinach in the bottom of the casserole. Arrange the fish fillets on top. Spread the cheese mixture on top of the fillets.

Bake for about 45 minutes, or until the edges are browned.

NOTES

This recipe works well with chicken too.

NUTRITIONAL DATA

597 calories, 30g fat, 497mg sodium, 1g fiber, 3g carbohydrates, 29g protein

2g net carbs, 2% carbs, 29% protein, 69% fat

SALMON WITH CREAMY DILL SAUCE

NUT-FREE | EGG-FREE

PREP TIME: 5 minutes	**COOK TIME:** 25 minutes
TOTAL TIME: 30 minutes	**SERVINGS:** 6

Salmon is so good, you typically don't need to add anything to it. But if you've gone keto, sometimes you need to add extra fat. What better source than a classic buttery cream sauce? It adds elegance to this simple baked salmon dish.

2 tablespoons butter

2 pounds salmon fillets

¼ cup heavy cream

1 teaspoon Dijon mustard

½ teaspoon dried dill or 1½ teaspoons fresh

Preheat the oven to 375°F. Butter a rimmed sheet pan or casserole dish.

Place the fish fillets in the buttered pan. In a bowl, mix together the cream, mustard, and dill. Pour over the fish.

Bake for 20 to 25 minutes, until the fish flakes in the center.

NUTRITIONAL DATA

283 calories, 17g fat, 113mg sodium, 0g fiber, 0g carbohydrates, 30g protein

0g net carbs, 0% carbs, 41% protein, 59% fat

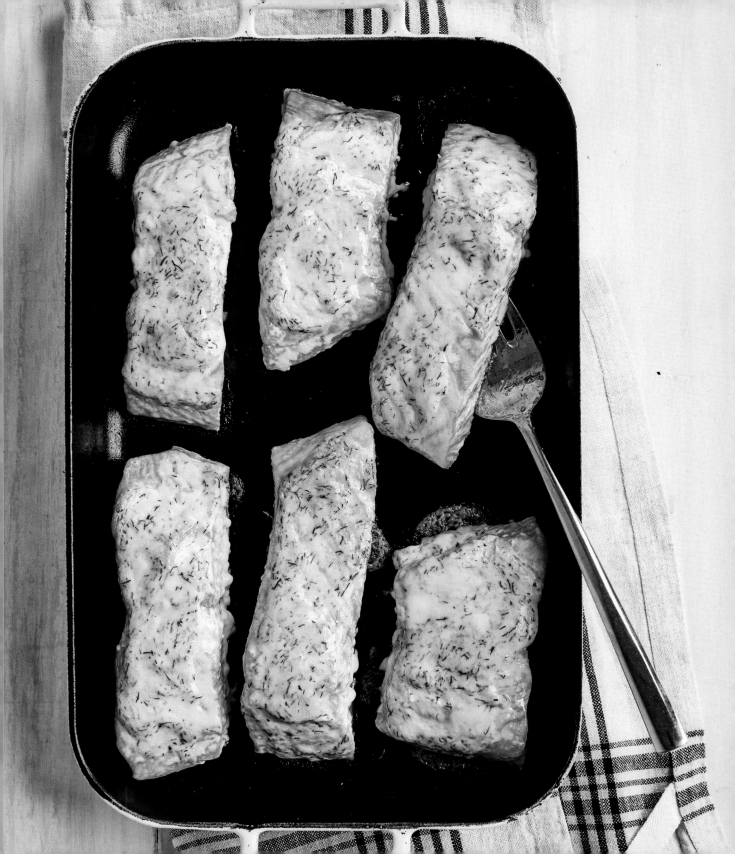

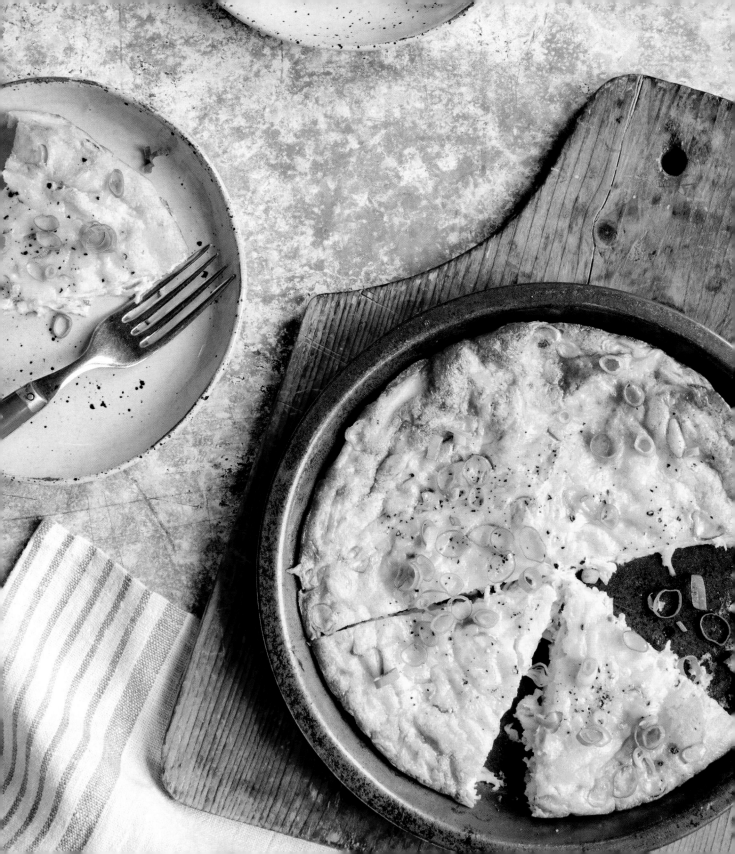

CRAB QUICHE

NUT-FREE

PREP TIME: 10 minutes
COOK TIME: 1 hour
TOTAL TIME: 1 hour, 10 minutes
SERVINGS: 6

Impress your friends next time you're invited to a potluck brunch with this crustless quiche with lump crabmeat. It whips up in just 10 minutes with only five main ingredients.

6 large eggs

1¼ cups heavy cream

12 ounces canned crabmeat

8 ounces shredded Swiss cheese

½ cup sliced green onions

½ teaspoon salt

Dash black pepper

NOTES

Cheddar cheese or other cheeses can be used instead of Swiss.

NUTRITIONAL DATA

427 calories, 33g fat, 823mg sodium, 0g fiber, 4g carbohydrates, 27g protein

4g net carbs, 4% carbs, 26% protein, 71% fat

Preheat the oven to 350°F.

In a large bowl, beat together the eggs and heavy cream. Stir in the crabmeat, cheese, onion, salt, and black pepper. Pour into a 9-inch deep-dish pie pan or a slightly larger-size pie pan.

Bake for 55 to 60 minutes, or until set.

SHRIMP SCAMPI

NUT-FREE | EGG-FREE

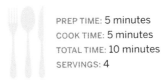

PREP TIME: 5 minutes
COOK TIME: 5 minutes
TOTAL TIME: 10 minutes
SERVINGS: 4

If you ordered shrimp scampi in an Italian restaurant without noodles, they'd probably think you're crazy. Well, let them have the belly-bloating carbs; you and I can relish the protein, savory spices, and healthy fat. Add zucchini noodles if you absolutely need something noodle-y.

4 tablespoons butter

3 large cloves garlic, minced

½ lemon

¼ teaspoon dried oregano

½ teaspoon salt

Dash black pepper

24 ounces frozen medium shrimp (cooked, shelled, and deveined), thawed

Chopped fresh parsley (optional), for garnish

Lemon slices (optional), for garnish

NOTES

For a complete meal, use this as a topping for spiralized zucchini or spaghetti squash.

NUTRITIONAL DATA

279 calories, 13g fat, 923mg sodium, 0g fiber, 2g carbohydrates, 35g protein

2g net carbs, 3% carbs, 53% protein, 44% fat

In a medium pot over low heat, combine the butter, garlic, juice from the lemon half, and oregano. Season with the salt and black pepper. Heat until the butter is melted.

Add the shrimp to the pot and coat completely with the butter mixture. Raise the heat to medium and cooking, stirring occasionally, until the shrimp is heated through, 4 to 5 minutes.

Serve with parsley sprinkled on top and lemon slices for garnish, if desired.

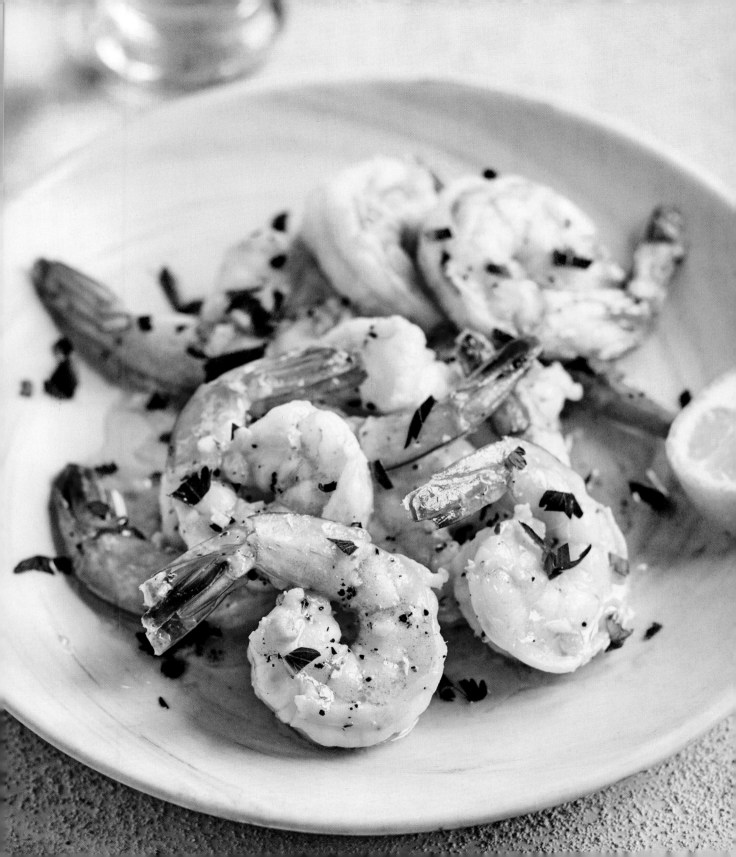

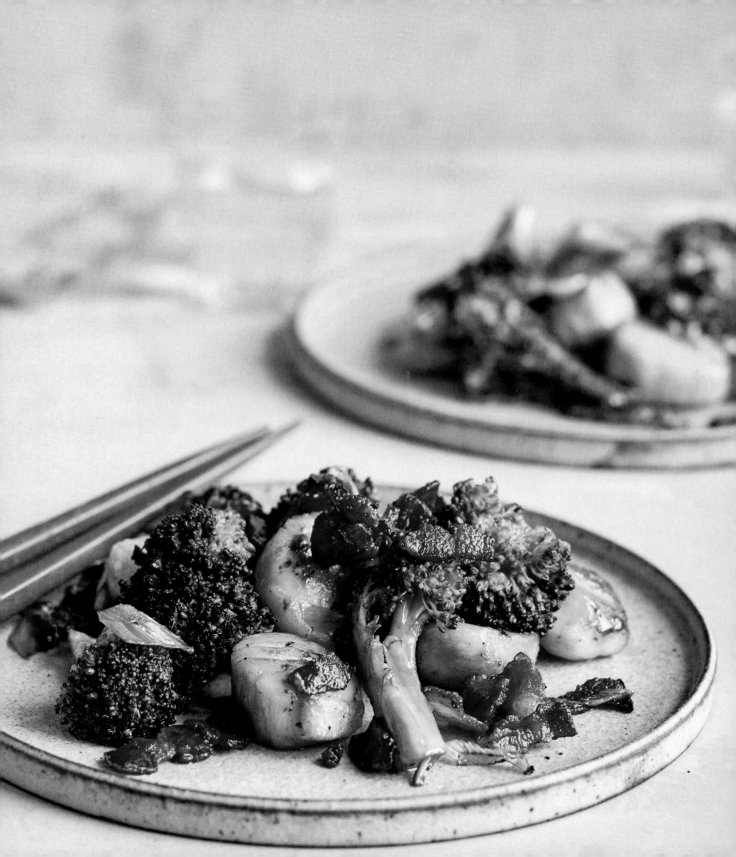

STIR-FRIED SCALLOPS

DAIRY-FREE | NUT-FREE | EGG-FREE | PALEO, AIP

PREP TIME: 10 minutes
COOK TIME: 20 minutes
TOTAL TIME: 30 minutes
SERVINGS: 3

A simple starch-free scallop stir-fry with bacon and broccoli. It's a dish that's sure to be a winner at get-togethers with friends or a quick family dinner at home.

6 ounces scallops

1½ tablespoons coconut aminos

6 slices bacon, cut into ½-inch pieces

3 green onions, sliced on an angle

6 ounces broccoli florets

If using large sea scallops, cut them into smaller halves. Place the scallops in a bowl. Stir in the coconut aminos to coat and let sit in the refrigerator until needed.

In a large skillet over medium heat, cook the bacon, stirring, until crisp, 6 to 8 minutes. Remove the bacon from the grease and set aside.

Add the scallops, green onions, and broccoli to the hot bacon grease. Cook over medium heat, stirring, until the scallops are fully cooked and the broccoli is tender, 3 to 5 minutes.

Stir in the bacon just before serving.

NUTRITIONAL DATA

251 calories, 17g fat, 1036mg sodium, 1g fiber, 7g carbohydrates, 15g protein

6g net carbs, 10% carbs, 25% protein, 65% fat

GARLICKY STEAMED MUSSELS

PREP TIME: 5 minutes
COOK TIME: 15 minutes
TOTAL TIME: 20 minutes
SERVINGS: 4

DAIRY-FREE | NUT-FREE | EGG-FREE | PALEO, AIP

Mussels are an inexpensive seafood that taste gourmet when steamed in a garlic broth. Serve them as an appetizer or to top spiralized vegetables.

2 pounds mussels

3 tablespoons extra-virgin olive oil

¼ cup chopped fresh parsley

4 cloves garlic, minced

½ cup Slow-Cooked Roasted Bone Broth (page 26)

½ teaspoon salt

Dash black pepper (omit for AIP)

Wash the mussels and clean by removing any barnacles and beards.

Heat the oil in a large skillet over medium-high heat. Add the parsley and garlic and cook, stirring, for 30 seconds to a minute. Add the mussels, broth, salt, and black pepper. Reduce the heat to medium, cover, and cook for about 10 minutes. Throw out any mussels with unopened shells.

NUTRITIONAL DATA

199 calories, 13g fat, 441mg sodium, 0g fiber, 5g carbohydrates, 14g protein

5g net carbs, 10% carbs, 29% protein, 61% fat

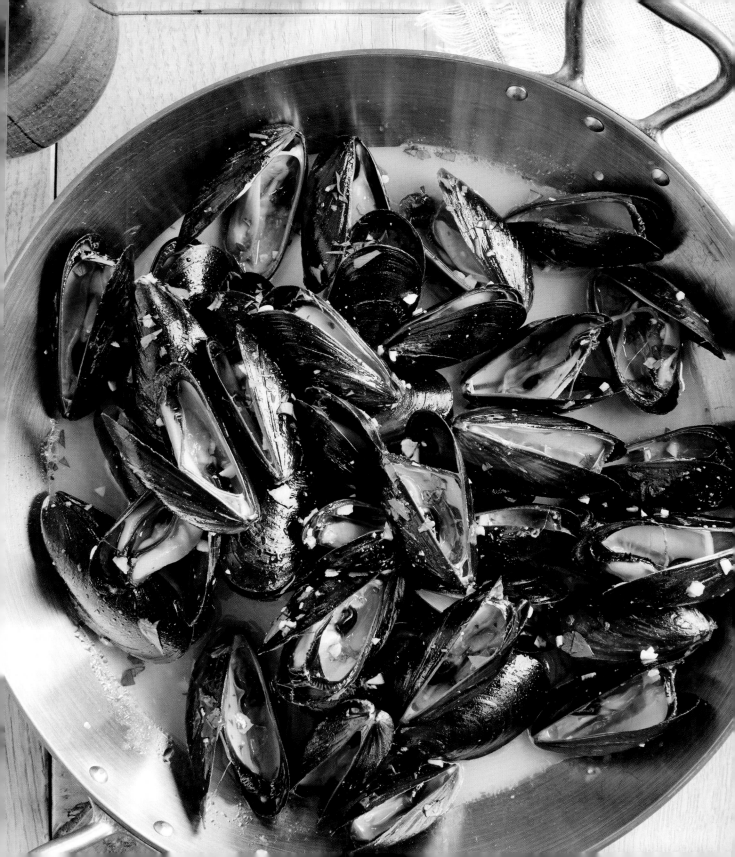

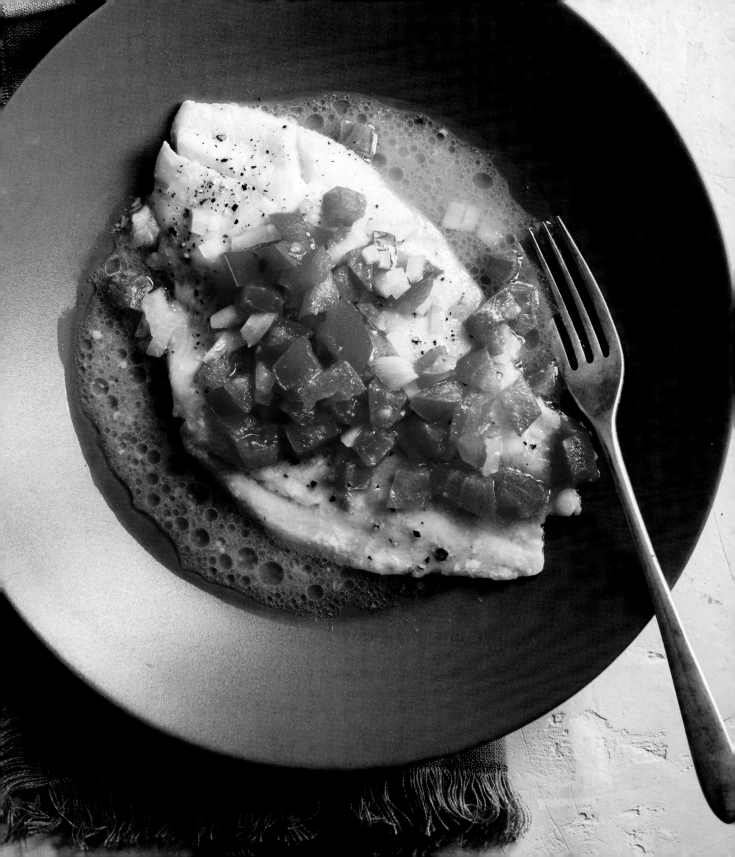

BAKED FLOUNDER WITH TOMATO

PREP TIME: 10 minutes
COOK TIME: 20 minutes
TOTAL TIME: 30 minutes
SERVINGS: 4

NUT-FREE | EGG-FREE

When you cook the flounder in a foil pouch, you'll feel like a grill master even though you're baking the fish. The foil seals in moisture and steams the fish, making it super juicy and tender.

1½ pounds flounder fillets

1 teaspoon salt

⅛ teaspoon black pepper

1 tomato, diced

¼ cup chopped onion

1 tablespoon chopped fresh basil

4 tablespoons butter

Lemon, for garnish

NOTES

The foil pouches can also be cooked on the grill.

NUTRITIONAL DATA

229 calories, 14g fat, 605mg sodium, 0g fiber, 2g carbohydrates, 21 g protein

2g net carbs, 4% carbs, 39% protein, 58% fat

Preheat the oven to 425°F.

Season each fillet with the salt and black pepper. Place each fillet on a piece of foil. Top each with some of the tomato, onion, and basil. Dot on the butter. Wrap the foil around each fillet to enclose. Place the foil pouches on a sheet pan.

Bake for 15 to 20 minutes, until the fish flakes easily with fork.

BALSAMIC HALIBUT

DAIRY-FREE | NUT-FREE | EGG-FREE | PALEO, AIP

PREP TIME: 5 minutes
COOK TIME: 20 minutes
TOTAL TIME: 25 minutes
SERVINGS: 3

Balsamic isn't just for drizzling on salads and strawberries. If you've never had it drizzled on fish, you're in for a tasty surprise! Olive oil adds some fat and sage provides a bolder taste.

2 tablespoon extra-virgin olive oil

1 tablespoon balsamic vinegar

½ teaspoon ground sage

¾ teaspoon salt

Dash black pepper (omit for AIP)

1 pound halibut fillets

Preheat the oven to 400°F. Coat the bottom of a sheet pan with the olive oil. Add the balsamic vinegar, sage, salt, and black pepper and blend well. Coat the fish fillets on all sides with the oil and vinegar mixture.

Cover the pan with foil. Bake until the fish is almost done, about 15 minutes. Remove the foil and bake until the fish flakes easily, about 5 minutes more.

NOTES

Flounder, cod, or wild striped bass fillets are great substitutes for the halibut.

You can also marinate the fish in the seasoned vinegar and oil mixture for 2 to 4 hours in the fridge before baking.

NUTRITIONAL DATA

224 calories, 11g fat, 104mg sodium, 0g fiber, 0g carbohydrates, 28g protein

0g net carbs, 0% carbs, 53% protein, 47% fat

TUNA CASSEROLE

NUT-FREE | EGG-FREE

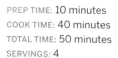

PREP TIME: 10 minutes
COOK TIME: 40 minutes
TOTAL TIME: 50 minutes
SERVINGS: 4

Tuna casserole has been a classic dish for over a hundred years. But this modern version omits the blood-sugar-spiking noodles and peas. Who needs those when you've got a creamy cheese sauce that satisfies both hunger and the taste buds?

1 tablespoon extra-virgin olive oil or butter, plus more for greasing

1 clove garlic, minced

1 cup heavy cream

1½ cups grated Parmesan cheese

Salt and black pepper

2 (5-ounce) cans tuna, drained

10 ounces frozen chopped spinach, thawed and drained

Chopped fresh parsley (optional), for garnish

Preheat the oven to 375°F. Lightly grease a casserole dish with some olive oil or butter.

Heat the oil or butter in a pot over medium-low heat. Add the garlic and cook, stirring, until golden, 1 to 2 minutes. Add the heavy cream and ½ cup water and cook, stirring, for about 5 minutes. Whisk in 1 cup of the Parmesan cheese and add salt and black pepper to taste.

Stir in the tuna and spinach. Raise the heat to medium-high and cook, stirring frequently, until just bubbling.

Spoon the tuna-and-spinach mixture into the prepared casserole dish. Sprinkle on the remaining ½ cup Parmesan cheese. Bake for 20 to 30 minutes, until bubbling. Garnish with parsley, if desired.

NOTES

Wilted fresh spinach can be used instead of frozen.

NUTRITIONAL DATA

466 calories, 36g fat, 851mg sodium, 2g fiber, 6g carbohydrates, 31g protein

4g net carbs, 3% carbs, 27% protein, 70% fat

BUTTER FISH

NUT-FREE | EGG-FREE

PREP TIME: 5 minutes
COOK TIME: 20 minutes
TOTAL TIME: 25 minutes
SERVINGS: 4

You don't need much to make the flavor of cod or flounder pop. Just add a little butter, salt, and pepper and a squirt of lemon. Keeping it simple in the kitchen is the way to go!

1 stick (4 ounces) salted butter

1 pound cod or flounder fillets

¾ teaspoon salt

Dash black pepper

1 lemon

½ teaspoon seafood seasoning

Preheat the oven to 400°F. Dot the butter over the bottom of a rimmed sheet pan.

Season the fish with salt and black pepper. Place the fish fillets over the butter on the sheet pan and bake for 10 minutes.

Remove from the oven and baste the fish with the melted butter from the pan. Season both sides of the fish with the juice from the lemon and the seafood seasoning. Bake for another 10 minutes, or until the fish flakes easily.

NOTES

A vegan butter substitute like butter-flavored coconut oil is a great way to enjoy this recipe without dairy.

NUTRITIONAL DATA

285 calories, 25g fat, 611mg sodium, 1g fiber, 1g carbohydrates, 14 g protein

0g net carbs, 0% carbs, 20% protein, 80% fat

CREAMY CLAM SAUCE OVER ZOODLES

PREP TIME: 10 minutes
COOK TIME: 25 minutes
TOTAL TIME: 35 minutes
SERVINGS: 4

NUT-FREE | EGG-FREE

Have linguine with clam sauce, but hold the pasta! When you replace high-carb linguine with spiralized zucchini, you can enjoy the classic dish without guilt or bloat.

2 zucchini

2 tablespoons butter

4 cloves garlic

1 pound clam meat

½ cup heavy cream

½ teaspoon salt

Black pepper

Chopped fresh parsley (optional), for garnish

Spiralize the zucchini. Set aside.

Melt the butter in a saucepan over medium-high heat. Add the garlic and cook, stirring, until tender, 2 to 3 minutes. Add the clam meat and cook, stirring, for another 2 to 3 minutes.

Add ½ cup water and bring to a boil. Reduce the heat and simmer until the liquid is reduced by about a quarter, 7 to 10 minutes. Stir in the heavy cream and simmer until the desired thickness is reached, about 5 minutes.

Season with the salt and black pepper to taste. Stir in the zucchini noodles and cook until the zoodles are softened, about 2 minutes.

Garnish with parsley, if desired.

NOTES

For a dairy-free version, use olive oil in place of the butter and 1 cup nondairy milk in place of the heavy cream and water.

NUTRITIONAL DATA

203 calories, 17g fat, 566mg sodium, 1g fiber, 6g carbohydrates, 7g protein

5g net carbs, 10% carbs, 14% protein, 76% fat

"BREADED" FLOUNDER

PREP TIME: 10 minutes
COOK TIME: 25 minutes
TOTAL TIME: 35 minutes
SERVINGS: 3

Can you still enjoy breaded fish fillets on keto? Absolutely! Just use high-protein almond flour instead of regular bread crumbs to make them. It's a much healthier alternative to batter-fried fish.

3 flounder fillets or other white fish fillets (about 1 pound)

⅓ cup mayonnaise

½ cup blanched almond flour

¼ cup grated Parmesan cheese

1 teaspoon Italian seasoning

¾ teaspoon salt

Dash black pepper

Preheat the oven to 375°F. Line a rimmed sheet pan with parchment paper or a silicone baking mat.

Coat the fish fillets with the mayonnaise.

Blend the almond flour, Parmesan cheese, Italian seasoning, salt, and black pepper together on a plate. Press the fillets into the dry mix to coat, then place them on the prepared sheet pan.

Bake for about 25 minutes. The fish should flake easily with a fork when fully cooked.

NOTES

Garnish with chopped fresh parsley and serve with lemon wedges.

For a dairy-free breading, replace the Parmesan cheese with 2 tablespoons nutritional yeast.

NUTRITIONAL DATA

414 calories, 32g fat, 739mg sodium, 2g fiber, 4g carbohydrates, 26g protein

2g net carbs, 2% carbs, 26% protein, 72% fat

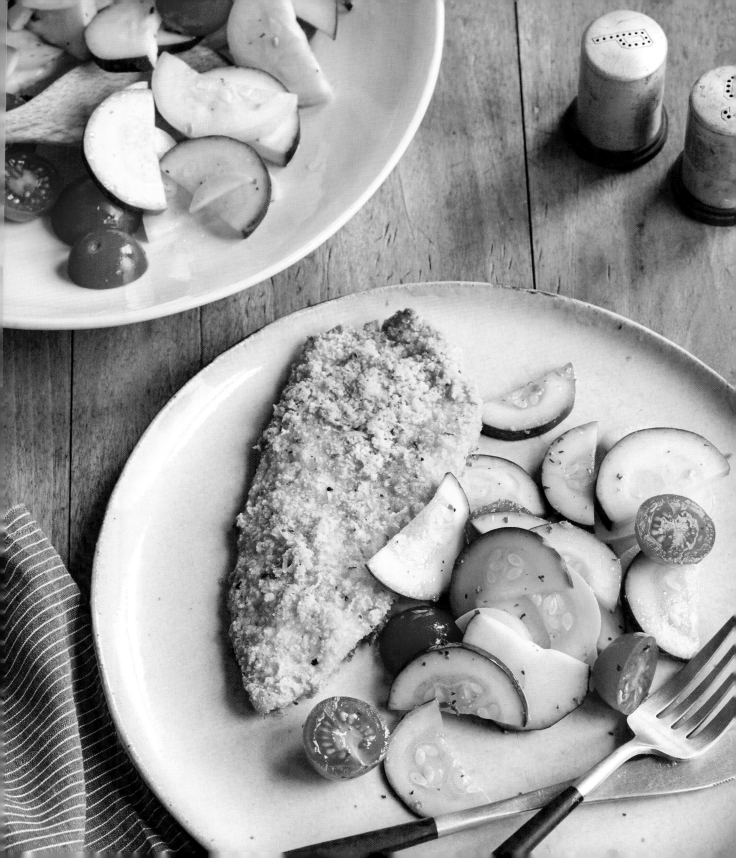

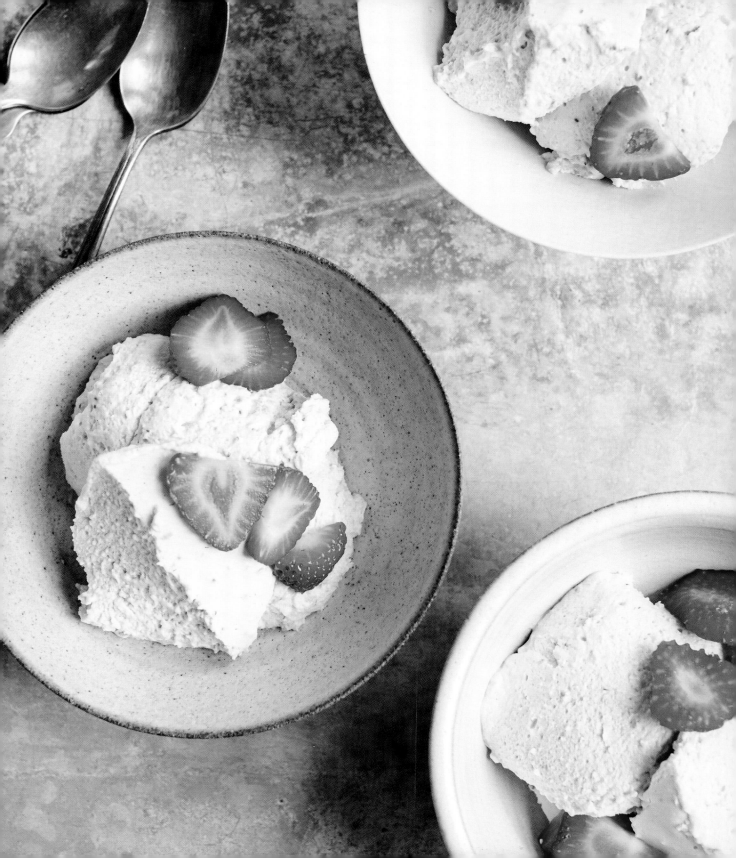

DESSERTS

Crustless Baked Cheesecake 186

Fluffy Strawberry Cream 189

Vanilla Custard Pudding 190

Raspberry-Cheese Muffins 191

Coconut Macaroons 192

Quick Ricotta Pudding 195

Chocolate Fudge Balls 195

No-Churn Vanilla Ice Cream 196

Baked Coffee Custard 198

Coconut Milk Pudding 199

Almond Butter Cookies 201

Chocolate Mousse 202

Almond Flour Cake 205

Almond Butter Cups 206

CRUSTLESS BAKED CHEESECAKE

PREP TIME: 5 minutes
COOK TIME: 30 minutes
TOTAL TIME: 35 minutes
SERVINGS: 4

NUT-FREE

Being able to enjoy creamy, high-fat cheesecake is one of the benefits of keto. And this is probably the easiest baked cheesecake ever! There's no crust to fuss with or slicing to worry about later. Serve with sliced strawberries or Strawberry Sauce (page 87) on top.

8 ounces cream cheese, softened

½ cup heavy cream

¼ cup monkfruit/erythritol granular sweetener

2 large eggs, at room temperature

2 teaspoons vanilla extract

Preheat the oven to 350°F.

Add the cream cheese, heavy cream, sweetener, eggs, and vanilla to a blender or food processor and blend until smooth, about 1 minute. Spread into an 8-inch round baking dish.

Bake for 25 to 30 minutes, until set. Let cool completely on a wire rack, about 30 minutes.

Chill for at least 2 hours before serving.

Use a small ice cream scoop to scoop out the cheesecake onto dessert plates or bowls.

NOTES

The ingredients blend easier when the cream cheese, cream, and eggs are set out at room temperature for an hour or two.

NUTRITIONAL DATA

334 calories, 32g fat, 224mg sodium, 0g fiber, 11g carbohydrates, 8g erythritol, 6g protein

3g net carbs, 4% carbs, 7% protein, 89% fat

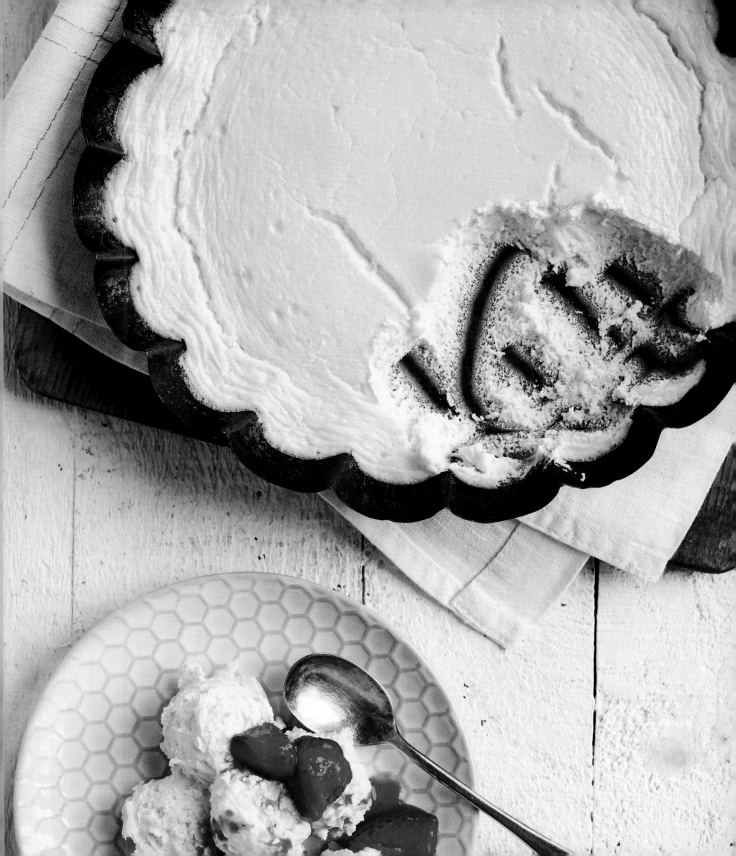

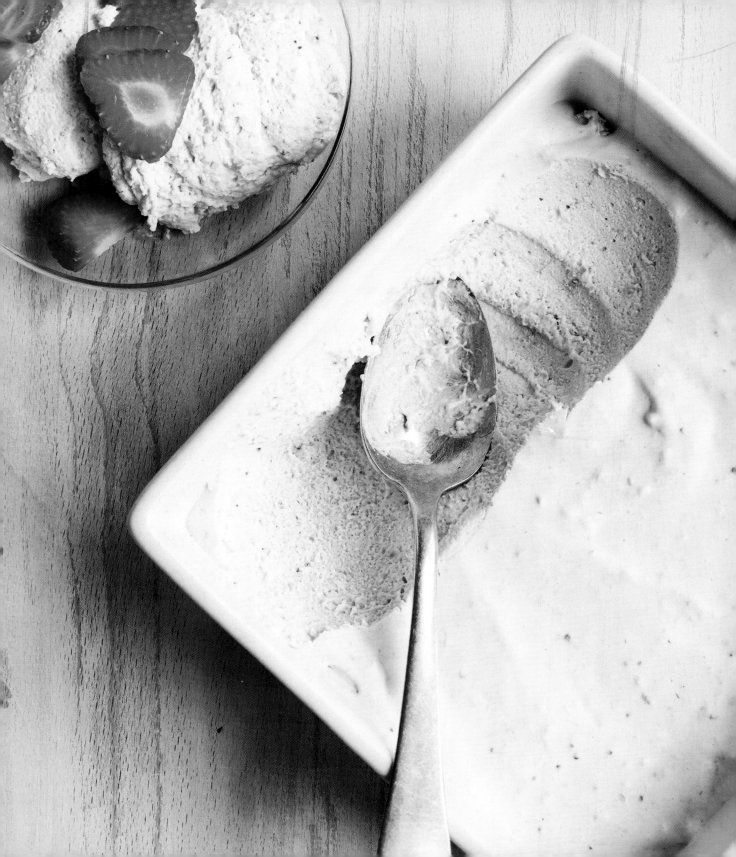

FLUFFY STRAWBERRY CREAM

PREP TIME: 10 minutes
COOK TIME: 5 minutes
TOTAL TIME: 15 minutes
SERVINGS: 6

NUT-FREE | EGG-FREE

A light and airy dessert bursting with fresh strawberry flavor. Not only is it low in carbs, it contains gelatin, which may help control blood sugar. It's sure to become a favorite keto dessert!

2 cups strawberries (1 pint)

¼ cup monkfruit/erythritol granular sweetener

1 tablespoon unflavored powdered gelatin

3 tablespoons boiling water

1½ cups heavy cream

1 teaspoon vanilla extract

Add the strawberries, sweetener, and ½ cup water to a medium saucepan over medium-low heat. Cook, stirring frequently, until the sweetener is dissolved. Transfer to a blender and puree. Set aside.

In a small cup or bowl, sprinkle the gelatin over 3 tablespoons cold water and let stand for a couple minutes to soften. Then add the boiling water and stir to dissolve the gelatin.

Add the cream to the bowl of a stand mixer fitted with the whisk attachment and whip while streaming in the dissolved gelatin and then the vanilla. Whip until it forms soft peaks. Gently fold in the strawberry puree. Beat for another 30 to 60 seconds. Chill for at least an hour before serving.

NOTES

For best results, use a chilled bowl to whip the cream.

Coconut cream can be used to make this dairy-free.

NUTRITIONAL DATA

226 calories, 22g fat, 25mg sodium, 0g fiber, 13g carbohydrates, 8g erythritol, 2g protein

5g net carbs, 6% carbs, 3% protein, 91% fat

VANILLA CUSTARD PUDDING

NUT-FREE

PREP TIME: 10 minutes
COOK TIME: 10 minutes
TOTAL TIME: 20 minutes
SERVINGS: 6

There's no need to add starch for a smooth, scrumptious, and creamy pudding. This cooked vanilla pudding is thickened with egg yolks and cream.

6 large egg yolks

¼ cup monkfruit/erythritol granular sweetener

8 ounces cream cheese

1¾ cups heavy cream

1 teaspoon vanilla extract

Fill the bottom of a double boiler with an inch of water and bring to a boil. In the top of the double boiler, beat together the egg yolks and sweetener. Place the top of the double boiler with the mixture in it over the boiling water. Reduce the heat to low and cook the egg yolk mixture, stirring constantly, for 8 to 10 minutes to thicken. Remove the mixture from the heat and beat in the cream cheese until well incorporated.

In a medium bowl, beat the heavy cream until stiff peaks form. Fold the whipped cream into the egg yolk mixture along with the vanilla.

Chill in one bowl or in single-serving dishes for at least 2 hours before serving. Store, covered, in the refrigerator for up to 1 week.

NUTRITIONAL DATA

428 calories, 43g fat, 156mg sodium, 0g fiber, 11g carbohydrates, 8g erythritol, 6g protein

3g net carbs, 3% carbs, 6% protein, 91% fat

RASPBERRY-CHEESE MUFFINS

PREP TIME: 10 minutes
COOK TIME: 20 minutes
TOTAL TIME: 30 minutes
SERVINGS: 12

NUT-FREE

Whether for dessert or an on-the-go breakfast in the car, these ultra-low-carb muffins will keep you going for hours. They are best served chilled and are similar to mini cheesecakes.

16 ounces cream cheese, softened

¼ cup monkfruit/erythritol granular sweetener

2 large eggs

½ teaspoon vanilla extract

¼ cup fresh raspberries

Preheat the oven to 350°F. Grease a 12-cup muffin tin or line it with silicone liners.

In a mixing bowl, beat the cream cheese with an electric mixer until smooth and creamy. Add the sweetener, eggs, and vanilla and beat until well blended. Fold in the raspberries.

Spoon the batter into the prepared muffin tin. Bake for about 20 minutes, or until set. Let cool in the muffin tin on a wire rack for 15 minutes, then transfer the muffins to the rack and let cool completely. Store, covered, in the refrigerator for up to a week.

NOTES

Using softened cream cheese allows for a smoother cream cheese mixture.

Other low-carb berries, sugar-free chocolate chips, or nuts can be used in place of the raspberries.

NUTRITIONAL DATA

141 calories, 13g fat, 131mg sodium, 0g fiber, 5g carbohydrates, 4g erythritol, 3g protein

1g net carbs, 3% carbs, 9% protein, 88% fat

COCONUT MACAROONS

PREP TIME: 10 minutes
COOK TIME: 12 minutes
TOTAL TIME: 22 minutes
SERVINGS: 20

DAIRY-FREE | NUT-FREE

Coconut macaroons are a flourless cookie loaded with sweetened coconut. However, low-carb sweetened coconut is impossible to find. That's why this recipe provides an easy method to sweeten dried coconut using a keto-friendly sweetener.

¾ cup monkfruit/erythritol granular sweetener

¾ teaspoon vanilla extract

¼ teaspoon salt

2 large eggs

3 cups unsweetened shredded coconut

Low-carb chocolate, melted (optional), for garnish

Preheat the oven to 350°F. Lightly spray a sheet pan with nonstick spray.

In a small saucepan, combine the sweetener, ⅓ cup water, the vanilla, and salt and bring to a boil over medium-high heat. Stir the resulting syrup and remove from the heat.

Combine the eggs and coconut in a food processor. Add the syrup and process for 1 to 2 minutes, until a dough is formed. Using an ice cream scoop with a release, place mounds of the dough about 1 inch apart on the prepared sheet pan.

Bake for about 8 minutes, then rotate the sheet pan 180 degrees and bake for an additional 4 minutes or until the cookies are light brown. Cool on a wire rack. Drizzle with melted chocolate, if desired.

NUTRITIONAL DATA

130 calories, 12g fat, 43mg sodium, 3g fiber, 11g carbohydrates, 7g erythritol, 1g protein

1g net carbs, 3.5% carbs, 3.5% protein, 93% fat

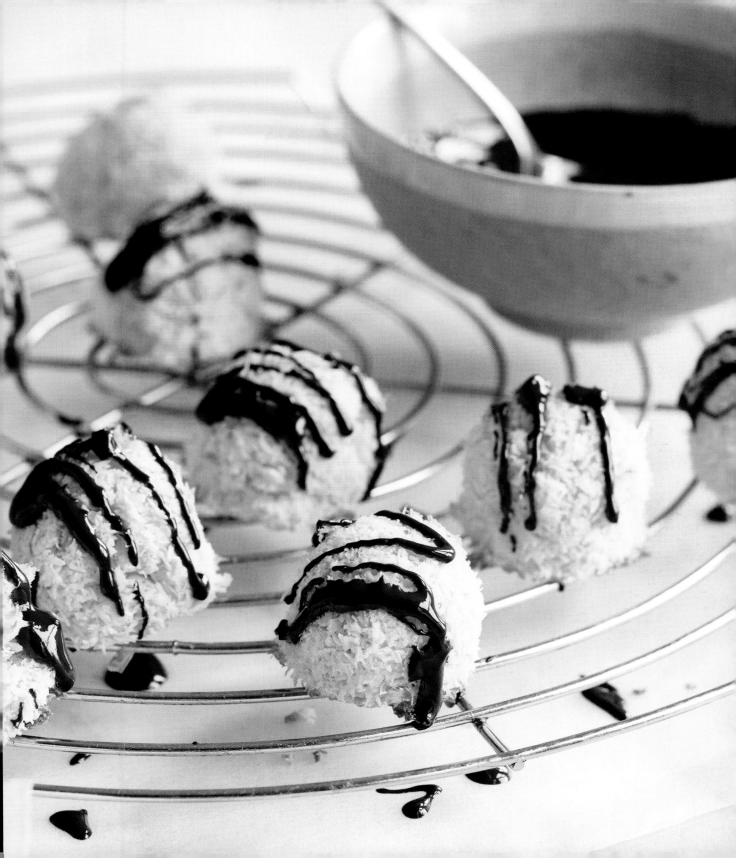

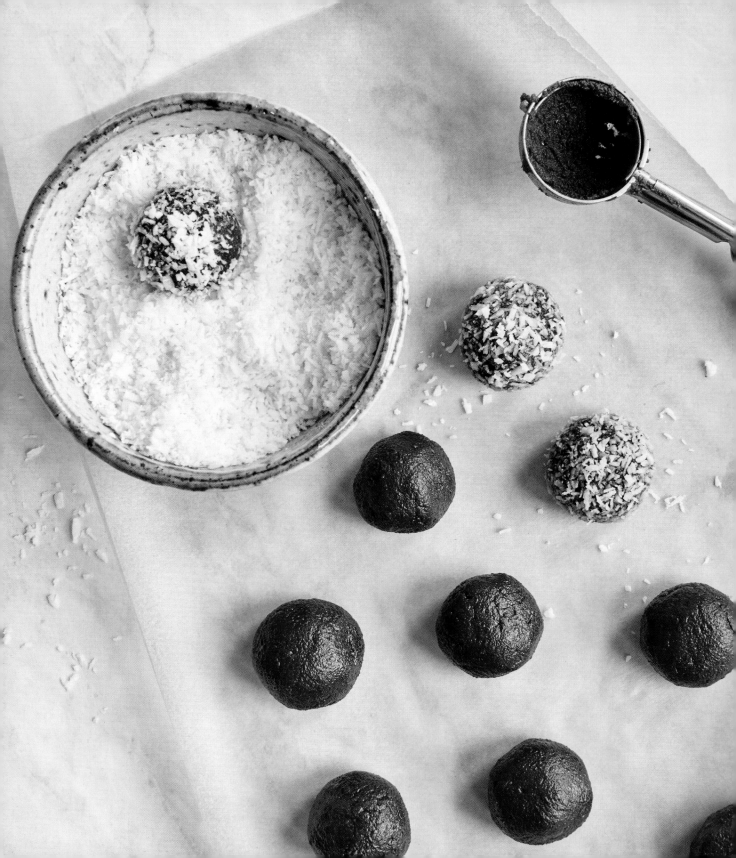

CHOCOLATE FUDGE BALLS

EGG-FREE

PREP TIME: 5 minutes   COOK TIME: 5 minutes
TOTAL TIME: 10 minutes   SERVINGS: 11

Since going low-carb, my cravings for sweets have been few. But when temptation does arise, I reach for my hidden stash of homemade fudge balls.

1 ounce unsweetened baking chocolate

¼ cup unsweetened almond butter

2 ounces cream cheese

2 teaspoons Swerve confectioners sweetener

1 teaspoon vanilla extract

In a saucepan over medium-low heat, combine the chocolate, almond butter, cream cheese, and sweetener and cook, stirring, until melted and well combined. Remove from the heat and stir in the vanilla.

Using your hands, form the mixture into tablespoon-size balls. Chill until firm.

NOTES

The balls can be rolled in unsweetened cocoa powder, unsweetened dried coconut, or chopped nuts for a prettier appearance and additional flavors.

NUTRITIONAL DATA

66 calories, 6g fat, 17mg sodium, 1g fiber, 3g carbohydrates, 1g erythritol, 1g protein

2g net carbs, 12% carbs, 6% protein, 82% fat

QUICK RICOTTA PUDDING

NUT-FREE | EGG-FREE

PREP TIME: 2 minutes   Total Time: 2 minutes
SERVINGS: 4

A mock rice pudding that's ready in only a couple minutes. And with just a few grams of net carbs, you can have a quick dessert any night, guilt-free!

1 cup cottage cheese

4 teaspoons plus 2 tablespoons monkfruit/ erythritol granular sweetener

¼ teaspoon ground cinnamon

1 cup heavy cream

Combine the cottage cheese, 4 teaspoons of the sweetener, and the cinnamon in a mixing bowl, then divide into four dessert cups. Refrigerate until ready to serve.

Chill a metal bowl for 15 to 20 minutes. Beat the heavy cream with the remaining 2 tablespoons sweetener in the chilled bowl until stiff peaks form. Serve with the whipped cream.

NUTRITIONAL DATA

257 calories, 24g fat, 213mg sodium, 0g fiber, 13g carbohydrates, 10g erythritol, 7g protein

3g net carbs, 5% carbs, 11% protein, 84% fat

NO-CHURN VANILLA ICE CREAM

PREP TIME: 10 minutes
COOK TIME: 10 minutes
TOTAL TIME: 20 minutes
SERVINGS: 10

NUT-FREE

No ice cream maker at home? No problem! Make this keto ice cream in the morning, and by the time you get home in the afternoon, it will be ready to enjoy. The texture is nice and creamy, just how you like it.

4 cups heavy cream

1 cup Swerve confectioners sweetener

2 large eggs, beaten

2½ teaspoons unflavored powdered gelatin (1 packet)

2 tablespoons vanilla extract

In a medium saucepan, combine the heavy cream, sweetener, eggs, gelatin, and vanilla. Set over medium heat and cook, stirring, until the mixture steams and the sweetener dissolves, 5 to 7 minutes.

Pour the mixture into a heat-safe bowl and cool in the refrigerator for about 1 hour. Once cooled, use an electric mixer to beat the cream mixture until soft peaks form.

Transfer to a freezer-safe container, cover, and freeze for at least 4 hours before serving.

NOTES

The mixture can be processed in an ice cream maker instead.

For a dairy-free version, use coconut cream in place of the heavy cream.

A fiber-based sweetener or allulose tends to freeze better than erythritol sweeteners, but more will be needed as it tends to be less sweet.

NUTRITIONAL DATA

351 calories, 36g fat, 50mg sodium, 0g fiber, 21g carbohydrates, 18g erythritol, 3g protein

3g net carbs, 4% carbs, 3% protein, 93% fat

VARIATIONS

Chocolate: Add 3 ounces chopped unsweetened chocolate and 2 tablespoons additional sweetener to the hot cream.

Coffee: Stir in 1 tablespoon instant coffee granules just before cooling.

Chocolate Chip: Stir in 3 ounces low-carb chocolate chips before freezing.

Toasted Coconut: Blend in 2 to 3 tablespoons toasted unsweetened shredded coconut before freezing.

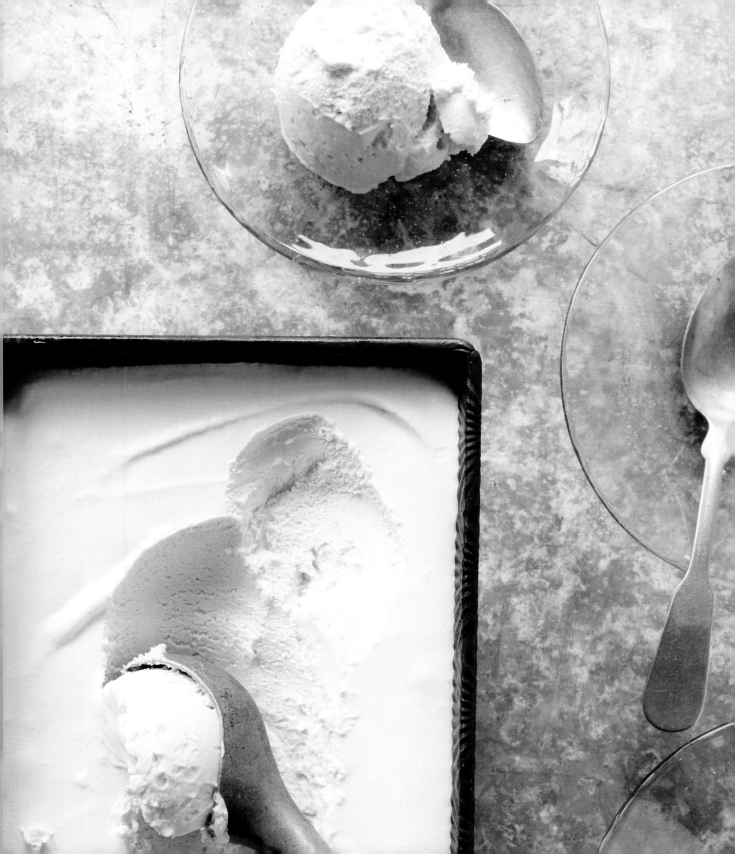

BAKED COFFEE CUSTARD

PREP TIME: 10 minutes
COOK TIME: 40 minutes
TOTAL TIME: 50 minutes
SERVINGS: 6

DAIRY-FREE

Need an afternoon pick-me-up? Save money and time skipping the Starbucks line by learning how to make this rich coffee treat. Dessert and coffee in one. Enough said! And enough servings for a whole workweek!

4 teaspoons instant coffee granules

4 large eggs

2 cups Almond Milk (page 210)

¼ cup monkfruit/erythritol granular sweetener

1 teaspoon vanilla extract

¼ teaspoon salt

Boiling water

Sweetened whipped cream (optional), for serving

Preheat the oven to 325°F.

In a small bowl, dissolve the instant coffee in 1 tablespoon hot water. Set aside.

In a medium bowl, lightly beat the eggs with the almond milk. Stir in the coffee, sweetener, vanilla, and salt.

Place six ramekins in a 9 × 13-inch casserole dish. Divide the mixture among the ramekins. Pour boiling water into the casserole dish to a depth of 1 inch.

Bake the custards for 30 to 40 minutes, until a toothpick or knife inserted into the center of a custard comes out clean. Carefully remove the ramekins from the water bath and cool on a wire rack.

The custard can be served warm or chilled, topped with whipped cream, if desired.

NUTRITIONAL DATA

194 calories, 18g fat, 148mg sodium, 0g fiber, 10g carbohydrates, 8g erythritol, 5g protein

2g net carbs, 4% carbs, 11% protein, 85% fat

COCONUT MILK PUDDING

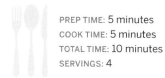

PREP TIME: 5 minutes
COOK TIME: 5 minutes
TOTAL TIME: 10 minutes
SERVINGS: 4

DAIRY-FREE | NUT-FREE | EGG-FREE

A stripped down, simple version of *maja blanca*, a popular dairy-free Filipino treat. Each bite transports you to Southeast Asia but without the carbs to worry about. Keep a few ready in the refrigerator for a quick snack.

2 teaspoons unflavored powdered gelatin

1 (13.5-ounce) can coconut milk

3 tablespoons monkfruit/erythritol granular sweetener

½ teaspoon vanilla extract

Toasted unsweetened shredded coconut (optional), for garnish

Add ¾ cup water to a small bowl or cup and stir the gelatin into it. Set aside.

Pour the coconut milk into a medium saucepan. Stir the sweetener and vanilla into the coconut milk. Bring the mixture to a boil, then stir in the gelatin mixture.

Pour into four dessert dishes or ramekins. Chill in the refrigerator for at least 4 hours. Serve topped with toasted coconut, if desired.

NOTES

The coconut cream will float to the top as it chills, creating two layers in the pudding.

NUTRITIONAL DATA

238 calories, 23g fat, 18mg sodium, 2 fiber, 10g carbohydrates, 5g erythritol, 4g protein

5g net carbs, 5% carbs, 7% protein, 88% fat

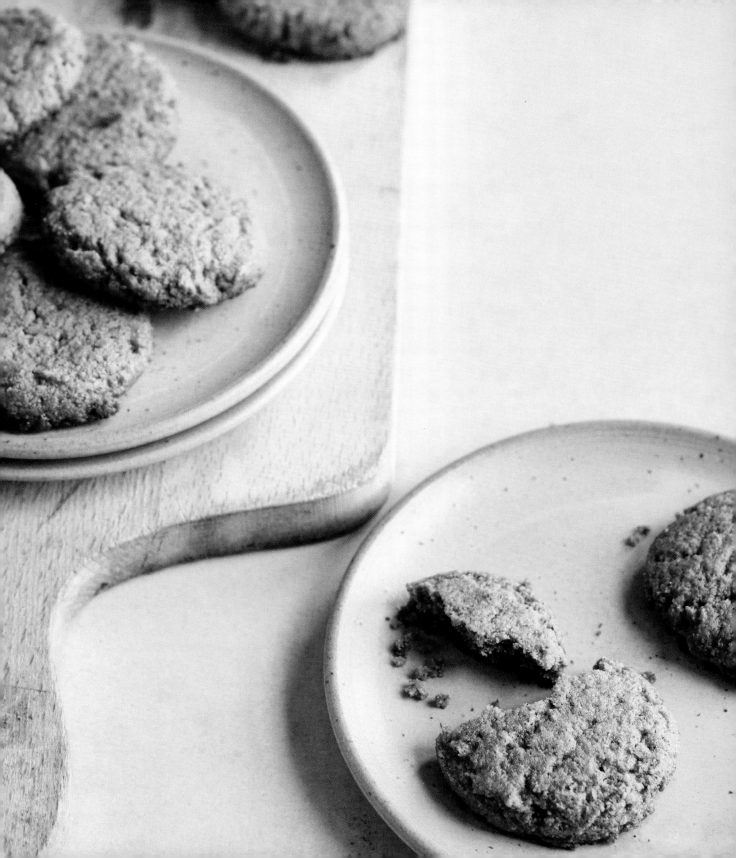

ALMOND BUTTER COOKIES

DAIRY-FREE

PREP TIME: 10 minutes
COOK TIME: 12 minutes
TOTAL TIME: 22 minutes
SERVINGS: 12 (2 cookies each)

Life is sweeter with cookies, even if there's only 3 grams of net carbs in each serving. Actually, life is way sweeter when you're able to enjoy cookies without the guilt, thanks to this keto-friendly version. Here, I keep it super simple by using a nut or seed butter as the base. And there are so many variations to try!

1 cup unsweetened almond butter

¼ cup monkfruit/erythritol granular sweetener

1 large egg

1 teaspoon baking soda

1 teaspoon vanilla extract

½ teaspoon salt

Preheat the oven to 350°F. Line two sheet pans with parchment paper or silicone baking mats.

In a large bowl, combine the almond butter with the sweetener. Add the egg, baking soda, vanilla, and salt and combine well.

Using a ice cream scoop or a spoon, form the dough into small balls and place on the prepared pans. Flatten each ball with the bottom of a glass or with a finger to the desired thickness. (Thinner will result in crispier cookies.)

Bake for 10 to 12 minutes, until the cookies are browned to desired crispness. Let them cool on the pan for 10 minutes, then transfer to a wire rack to cool completely.

NOTES

Add low-carb chocolate chips and or nuts. You can also dip half the cookie into melted low-carb chocolate.

These can be made with different nut or seed butters.

> **NUTRITIONAL DATA**
>
> 134 calories, 11g fat, 97mg sodium, 2g fiber, 7g carbohydrates, 4g erythritol, 4g protein
>
> 3g net carbs, 9% carbs, 13% protein, 78% fat

CHOCOLATE MOUSSE

PREP TIME: 10 minutes
TOTAL TIME: 10 minutes
SERVINGS: 4

NUT-FREE | EGG-FREE

Even if you were to eat two servings of my chocolate mousse (who eats just one serving?), you'd only consume 6 grams of net carbs. So the next time a chocolate craving gets the best of you, make this classic treat.

2½ teaspoons unflavored powdered gelatin (1 packet)

2 tablespoons boiling water

¼ cup monkfruit/erythritol granular sweetener

¼ cup unsweetened cocoa powder

1 cup heavy cream

1 teaspoon vanilla extract

In small cup, sprinkle the gelatin over 1 tablespoon cold water and let stand for 1 minute to soften. Add the boiling water and stir until the gelatin is completely dissolved and the mixture is clear. Cool slightly.

In a medium bowl, stir together the sweetener and cocoa powder. Add the heavy cream and vanilla.

Beat with an electric mixer on medium speed, scraping the bottom of the bowl occasionally if needed, until the mixture is thickened. Pour in the gelatin mixture and beat until well blended.

Spoon into four serving dishes and refrigerate for at least 2 hours before serving.

NOTES

Coconut cream can be used in place of heavy cream for a coconutty dairy-free version.

NUTRITIONAL DATA

223 calories, 22g fat, 26mg sodium, 1g fiber, 15g carbohydrates, 11g erythritol, 3g protein

3g net carbs, 5% carbs, 5% protein, 89% fat

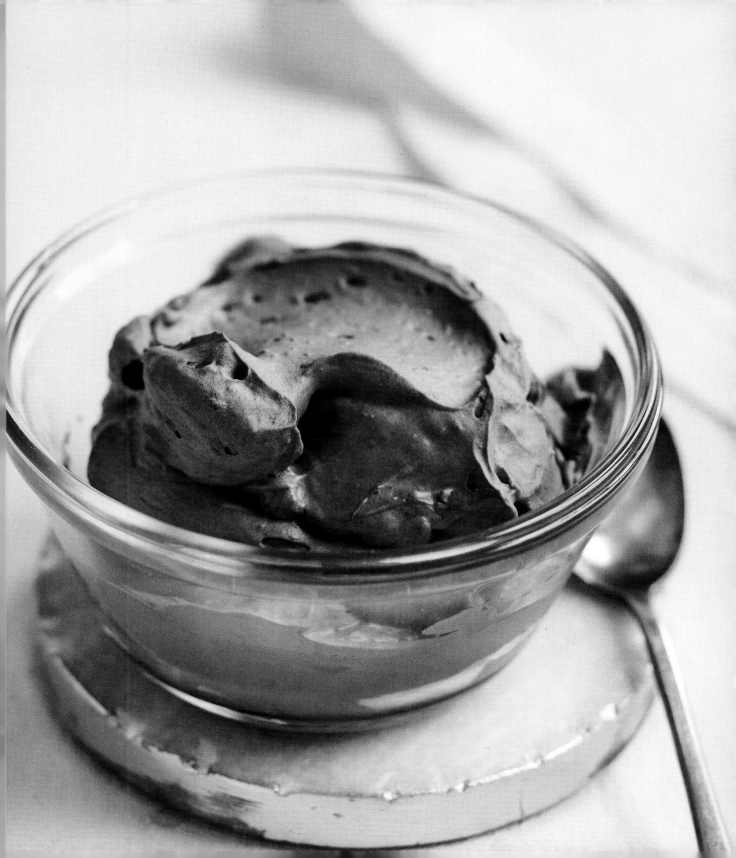

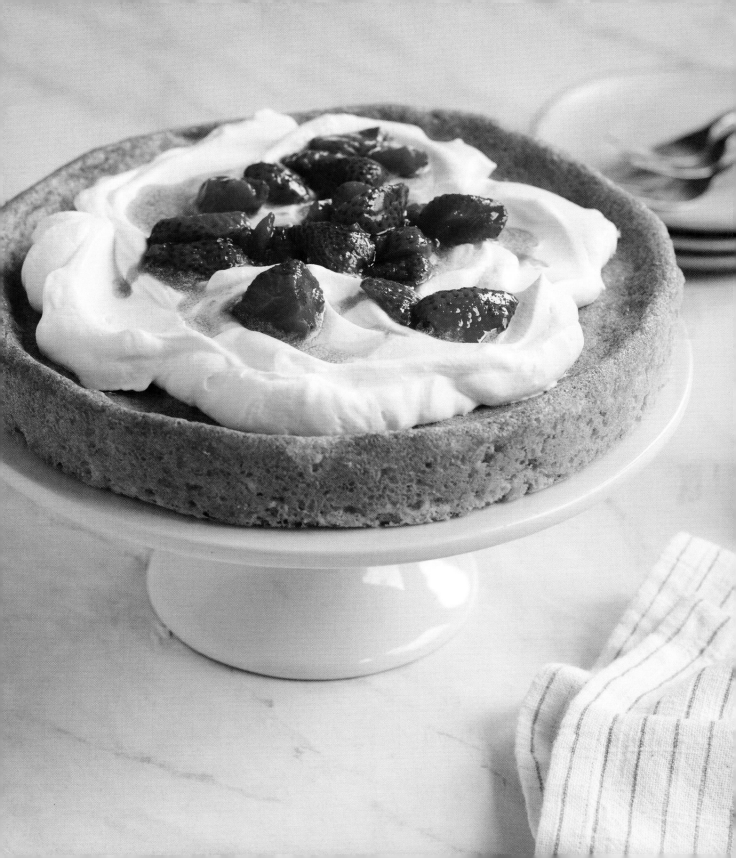

ALMOND FLOUR CAKE

DAIRY-FREE

PREP TIME: 10 minutes
COOK TIME: 15 minutes
TOTAL TIME: 25 minutes
SERVINGS: 8

A light and airy almond cake made without any dairy and just a hint of a crust-like texture to mirror the high-carb version. Dress it up with some Strawberry Sauce (page 87) and cream or a drizzle of Chocolate Sauce (page 87).

¾ cup blanched almond flour

1 teaspoon baking powder

⅛ teaspoon salt

3 large eggs, at room temperature

¼ cup monkfruit/erythritol granular sweetener

1 teaspoon vanilla extract

Preheat the oven to 325°F. Grease a 9-inch round pan or line the bottom with parchment paper.

In a medium bowl, combine the almond flour, baking powder, and salt.

In a large bowl using an electric mixer, beat the eggs and sweetener until the mixture is about 3 times the initial volume, 8 to 10 minutes. Beat in the vanilla, then fold in the almond flour mixture. Spread the batter into the prepared pan.

Bake for 20 to 25 minutes, until a cake tester or toothpick inserted into the center of the cake comes out clean. Let cool in the pan on a wire rack for at least 15 minutes before removing from pan.

NOTES

For a strawberry shortcake, serve with Strawberry Sauce (page 87) and whipped cream.

NUTRITIONAL DATA

84 calories, 6g fat, 60mg sodium, 1g fiber, 8g carbohydrates, 6g erythritol, 4g protein

2g net carbs, 6% carbs, 13% protein, 81% fat

ALMOND BUTTER CUPS

DAIRY-FREE | EGG-FREE | PALEO

PREP TIME: 15 minutes
COOK TIME: 15 minutes
TOTAL TIME: 30 minutes
SERVINGS: 8

I have to hide these cups; otherwise they will get devoured in a flash. They are great to have on hand to satisfy any chocolate bar cravings. And when made without sugar alcohol, the treat won't cause digestive issues.

¼ cup unsweetened almond butter

¼ cup coconut oil

2 ounces unsweetened baking chocolate

½ teaspoon vanilla extract

¼ teaspoon liquid stevia extract

Line eight wells of a mini-muffin pan with cupcake liners (or use silicone mini-muffin cups).

In a saucepan over low heat, combine the almond butter, coconut oil, and baking chocolate and cook, stirring, until melted and well combined, 10 to 15 minutes. Remove from the heat. Stir in the vanilla and stevia.

Divide the mixture among the prepared muffin cups. Chill to set and keep refrigerated or frozen.

NOTES

Using a sweetener that contains erythritol may make the chocolate crunchy, as the sweetener may not dissolve completely, so it's recommended to use either stevia or monkfruit extract in this recipe.

Other nut or seed butters can be used in the recipe as well, like peanut butter.

NUTRITIONAL DATA

142 calories, 14 fat, 2mg sodium, 1g fiber, 3g carbohydrates, 0g erythritol, 2g protein

2g net carbs, 6% carbs, 6% protein, 88% fat

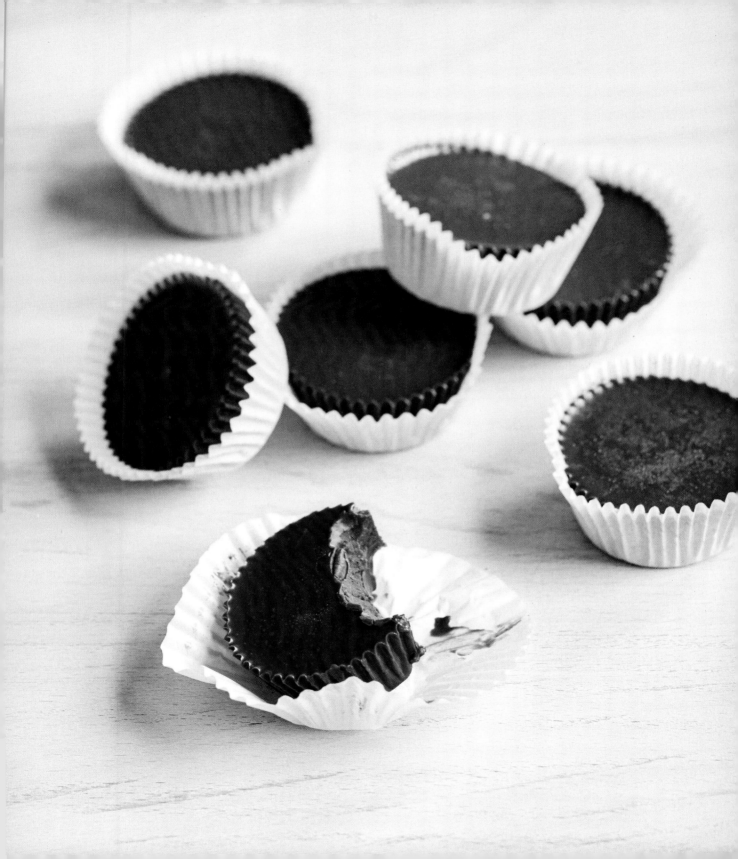

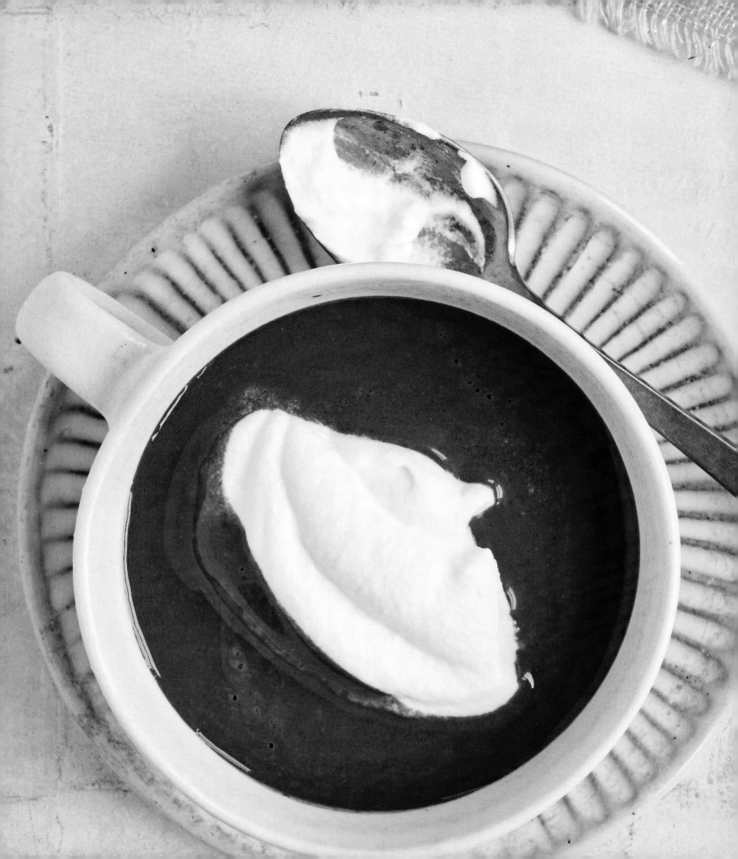

BEVERAGES

Keto Coffee or Tea 210
Almond Milk 210
Green Tea Smoothie 211
Raspberry Smoothie 211
Golden Milk 215
Hot Cocoa 215
Strawberry Milkshake 216
Strawberry Lemonade 216
Ginger-Turmeric Tea 218

KETO COFFEE OR TEA

DAIRY-FREE | NUT-FREE | EGG-FREE | PALEO

PREP TIME: 5 minutes TOTAL TIME: 5 minutes
SERVINGS: 1

A cup of joe or tea that's so creamy and frothy, it can take the place of eating breakfast if you're trying to reduce calories or gently wake up your digestion when you're intermittent fasting. Using MCT oil provides your brain and body with long-lasting fuel and balances the caffeine.

1¼ cups coffee or tea
1 tablespoon coconut oil, MCT oil, or butter
1 tablespoon canned coconut milk or butter
⅛ teaspoon ground cinnamon (optional)
1 scoop collagen (optional)

Add the coffee, coconut oil, coconut milk, cinnamon, and collagen, if using, to a tall mug. Blend together with a milk frother or spoon. Alternatively, use a blender to blend well.

NUTRITIONAL DATA

158 calories, 17g fat, 8mg sodium, 0g fiber, 0g carbohydrates, 0g protein

0g net carbs, 0% carbs, 0% protein, 100% fat

ALMOND MILK

DAIRY-FREE | EGG-FREE | PALEO

PREP TIME: 20 minutes SOAK TIME: 8 hours
TOTAL TIME: 8 hours, SERVINGS: 5
    20 minutes

This is how almond milk is supposed to taste: rich and nutty, not watered down. You may never buy commercial almond milk again!

1 cup unsalted raw almonds
4 to 5 cups water, preferably filtered
Pinch salt

Soak the almonds overnight in enough water to cover. Remove the skins and rinse.

Place the almonds, 4 to 5 cups water (less for thicker milk), and salt in a blender. Blend until smooth. Line a bowl with a double layer of cheesecloth or a clean thin dish towel and pour in the almond mixture. Gather the edges of the cheesecloth or towel and twist to squeeze out as much liquid as possible.

Pour the almond milk into a glass jar, seal, and store in the refrigerator for 5 to 7 days.

NOTES

Hazelnuts, macadamias, pecans, and walnuts can also be used. Pecans and walnuts only need about 4 hours of soaking.

NUTRITIONAL DATA

30 calories, 2g fat, 19mg sodium, 1g fiber, 2g carbohydrates, 1g protein

1g net carbs, 15% carbs, 15% protein, 70% fat

GREEN TEA SMOOTHIE

DAIRY-FREE | NUT-FREE | EGG-FREE | PALEO, AIP

PREP TIME: 5 minutes   TOTAL TIME: 5 minutes
SERVINGS: 4

Instead of a heavy breakfast, fill up with a double dose of high-antioxidant leafy green spinach and the healthy fats of creamy avocado. Or make this to stave off any cravings you may experience between lunch and dinner.

3 cups ice
2 cups (1.4 ounces) baby spinach
1½ cups strong brewed green tea
1 medium avocado, pitted
2 tablespoons lemon juice
20 drops liquid stevia extract

Combine the ice, spinach, green tea, avocado, lemon juice, and sweetener in a high-speed blender. Blend until smooth. Divide into four servings.

NOTES

I find stevia or monkfruit liquid sweeteners work best for smoothies, but 4 teaspoons of granular sweetener can be used instead.

NUTRITIONAL DATA

171 calories, 14g fat, 30mg sodium, 7g fiber, 10g carbohydrates, 2g protein

3g net carbs, 8% carbs, 6% protein, 86% fat

RASPBERRY SMOOTHIE

DAIRY-FREE | NUT-FREE | EGG-FREE | PALEO, AIP

PREP TIME: 5 minutes   TOTAL TIME: 5 minutes
SERVINGS: 2

Raspberries are a keto-friendly fruit, but they're even better for you when you combine them with a healthy fat like avocado. And even better than that is adding both of them to a creamy, nondairy, low-carb smoothie.

¼ cup frozen raspberries
1 medium avocado, pitted
Juice of one lemon
¼ teaspoon liquid stevia extract

Combine 1⅓ cups water, the raspberries, avocado, lemon juice, and stevia in a high-speed blender and blend until smooth. Divide into two equal servings. One can be enjoyed now and the other later!

NOTES

Any mix of frozen raspberries, blackberries, blueberries, and strawberries can be used. Strawberries don't have a strong red color, so a little beet powder can be added to hide the green.

NUTRITIONAL DATA

169 calories, 15g fat, 16mg sodium, 8g fiber, 10g carbohydrates, 2g protein

2g net carbs, 5% carbs, 5% protein, 89% fat

RASPBERRY SMOOTHIE (PAGE 211)

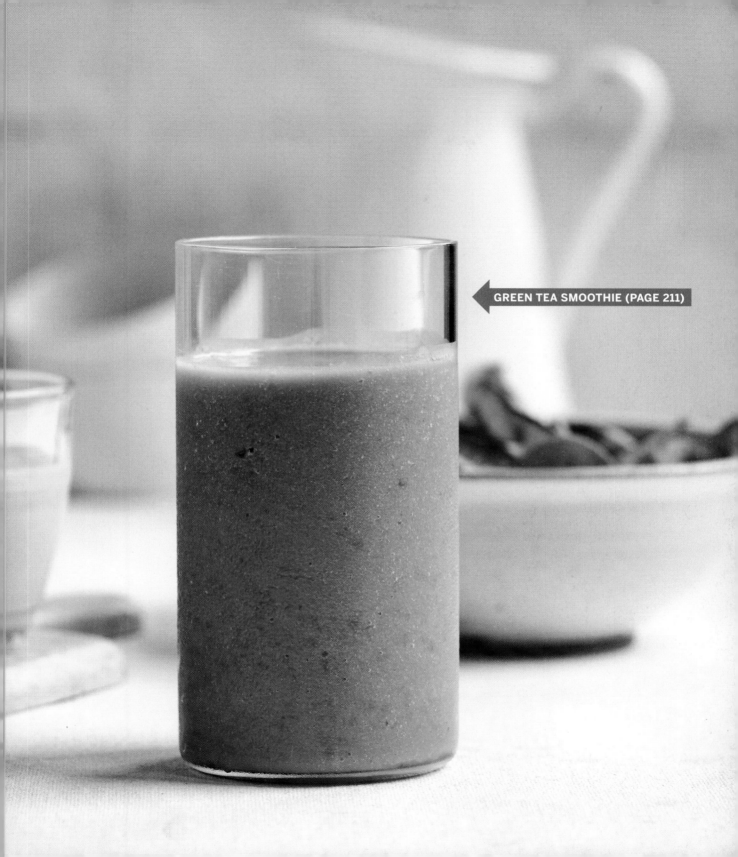

GREEN TEA SMOOTHIE (PAGE 211)

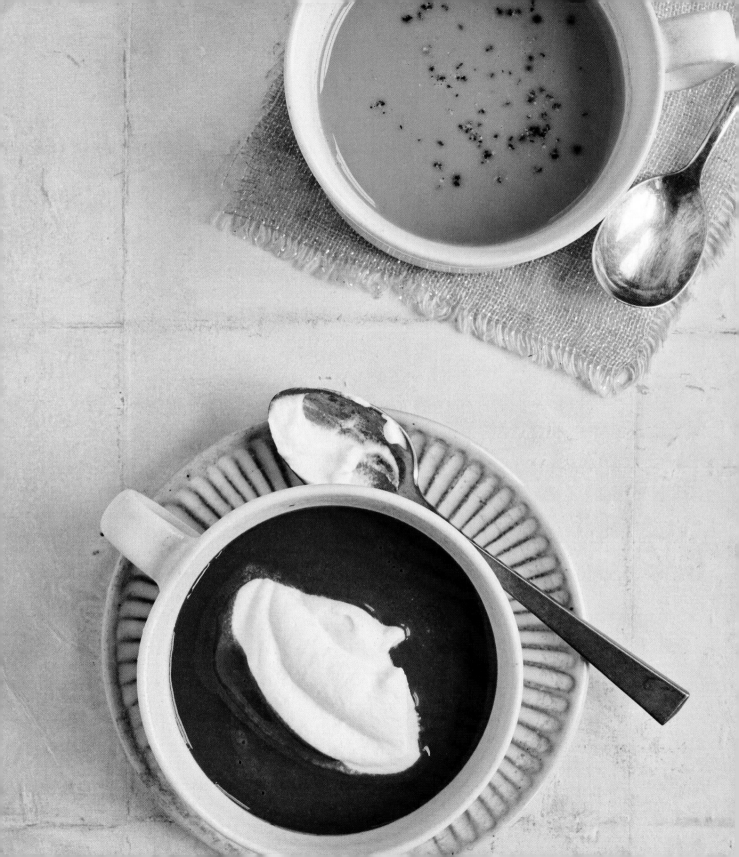

GOLDEN MILK

DAIRY-FREE | EGG-FREE | PALEO, AIP

PREP TIME: 5 minutes	COOK TIME: 15 minutes
TOTAL TIME: 20 minutes	SERVINGS: 1

Whether you serve it hot or cold, this is one of the tastiest and healthiest drinks on the planet, not to mention simple to make. Turmeric and ginger contain inflammation-fighting compounds. Drink this every day and your aches and pains may go away!

1 cup unsweetened almond milk or coconut milk beverage (if AIP)

1 teaspoon ground turmeric

½ teaspoon ground ginger

½ teaspoon ground cinnamon, plus more to taste

Pinch black pepper (omit for AIP)

5 drops liquid stevia extract (optional)

Combine the milk, turmeric, ginger, cinnamon, black pepper, and sweetener, if desired, in a small saucepan. Bring to a boil, then reduce the heat and simmer for 10 minutes. Top with additional cinnamon, if desired.

NOTES

Make sure you include the black pepper because without it, your body can't absorb the turmeric as well.

NUTRITIONAL DATA

49 calories, 3g fat, 326mg sodium, 2g fiber, 4g carbohydrates, 2g protein

2g net carbs, 18% carbs, 19% protein, 63% fat

HOT COCOA

DAIRY-FREE | EGG-FREE

PREP TIME: 5 minutes	COOK TIME: 10 minutes
TOTAL TIME: 15 minutes	SERVINGS: 2

Does a cocoa with almond milk and stevia compare with the sinfully delicious regular high-sugar and dairy version? And more than taste, does drinking it stir up images of cozy nights in front of the fire and building snowmen? The answers: yes and yes!

3 tablespoons unsweetened cocoa powder

1½ tablespoons monkfruit/erythritol granular sweetener, or to taste

2 cups Almond Milk (page 210)

½ teaspoon vanilla extract

Unsweetened whipped cream (optional), for serving

Mix the cocoa and sweetener in a small bowl.

In a small saucepan, whisk together the almond milk and the cocoa mixture. Heat over medium-high heat, stirring, for 5 to 7 minutes, until the cocoa is steaming and the desired temperature is reached.

Remove from the heat and stir in the vanilla.

Divide between two mugs. Top with whipped cream, if desired.

NUTRITIONAL DATA

55 calories, 4g fat, 327mg sodium, 3g fiber, 17g carbohydrates, 13g erythritol, 3g protein

1g net carbs, 8% carbs, 23% protein, 69% fat

STRAWBERRY MILKSHAKE

EGG-FREE

PREP TIME: 5 minutes TOTAL TIME: 5 minutes
SERVINGS: 1

A drive-thru-quality milkshake without all the calories and carbs. It's thick and satisfying but won't go straight to your midsection or spike your blood sugar.

1 cup Almond Milk (page 210)
½ cup ice
¼ cup frozen strawberries
1 ounce cream cheese
5 drops liquid stevia extract
⅛ teaspoon vanilla extract

Combine the milk, ice, strawberries, cream cheese, sweetener, and vanilla in a high-speed blender and blend until smooth, 15 to 30 seconds. Pour in to a tall glass.

NOTES

Top with whipped cream, if desired.

Adding collagen or whey protein can turn this shake into a light meal.

NUTRITIONAL DATA

145 calories, 13g fat, 412mg sodium, 1g fiber, 10g carbohydrates, 5g erythritol, 3g protein

4g net carbs, 11% carbs, 8% protein, 81% fat

STRAWBERRY LEMONADE

DAIRY-FREE | NUT-FREE | EGG-FREE | PALEO, AIP

PREP TIME: 10 minutes TOTAL TIME: 10 minutes
SERVINGS: 8

Got kids? They're gonna love this healthy and refreshing drink. It's as tasty as a juice box, but without the high amount of sugar. You may not want to share!

1½ cups strawberries, sliced
¾ cup lemon juice
1½ teaspoons liquid stevia extract (more or less to taste)
Ice

Combine the strawberries and lemon juice in a blender and blend until smooth.

Pour the fruit mixture into 2-quart pitcher. Stir in 5 cups water and the stevia. Add ice to fill the pitcher. Serve cold.

NUTRITIONAL DATA

14 calories, 1g fat, 8mg sodium, 1g fiber, 4g carbohydrates, 1g protein

3g net carbs, 48% carbs, 16% protein, 36% fat

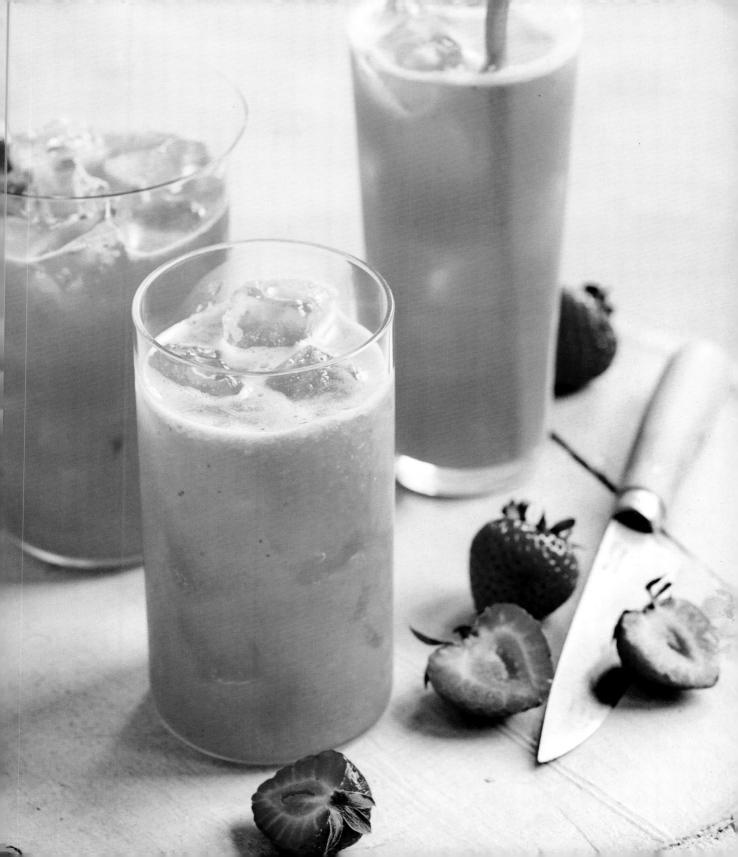

GINGER-TURMERIC TEA

PREP TIME: 5 minutes
COOK TIME: 15 minutes
TOTAL TIME: 20 minutes
SERVINGS: 2

DAIRY-FREE | NUT-FREE | EGG-FREE | PALEO, AIP

Turmeric and ginger are both known for their anti-inflammatory and antioxidant properties. Combining the two spices into a tea is not only flavorful but provides amazing health benefits.

1½ tablespoons chopped fresh ginger

½ teaspoon ground turmeric

¼ teaspoon ground cinnamon

Dash black pepper (omit for AIP)

10 drops liquid stevia extract (optional)

Lemon slices (optional, for garnish)

Bring 2 cups water to a boil in a medium saucepan. Add the ginger, turmeric, cinnamon, and black pepper. Reduce the heat and simmer for about 10 minutes.

Strain the ginger out, if desired, and pour into large mugs. Add sweetener, if desired. Top each with a slice of lemon for garnish and flavor, if desired.

NOTES

Dried stevia leaves work well as a sweetener in tea.

NUTRITIONAL DATA

6 calories, 0g fat, 13mg sodium, 0g fiber, 1g carbohydrates, 0g protein

1g net carbs, 100% carbs, 0% protein, 0% fat

INDEX

Note: Page references in *italics* refer to photos of recipes.

A

Almonds
  Almond Asparagus, 111, *113*
  Almond Butter Cookies,
    200, 201
  Almond Butter Cups, 206,
    207
  Almond Cheese, 72, *75*
  Almond Flour Bread, 70, *71*
  Almond Flour Cake, *204*,
    205
  Almond Flour Pancakes,
    2, 3
  Almond Milk, 210
  Coconut–Almond Butter
    Bars, *12*, 13
Appetizers and snacks,
    69–83
  Almond Cheese, 72, *75*
  Almond Flour Bread, 70, *71*
  Avocado Deviled Eggs,
    74, 79
  Cheese Ball, 78
  Mexican Cheese Dip, 73
  Nutty Crackers, *75*, 76
  Seasoned Tortilla Chips,
    80, *81*
  Sour Cream and Onion Dip,
    82, 83
  Stuffed Cucumber Slices, 77
Asparagus, Almond, 111, *113*
Asparagus, Ginger Beef and,
    148, *149*

Avocados
  Avocado Deviled Eggs,
    74, 79
  Avocado Dressing, 86, *91*
  Avocado Mayonnaise, 89
  Creamy Avocado Soup,
    36, 37
  Spinach-Tomato-Avocado
    Omelet, *6*, 7

B

Baby Kale Salad, 58
Baby Vegetable Mixed Salad,
    50, *51*
Bacon
  Bacon-Egg Cups, 10
  Breakfast Burrito, 20
  Broccoli and Cheese
    Stuffed Chicken, *122*, 123
  Fried Cabbage with Bacon,
    102, *103*
  Roasted Brussels with
    Bacon Soup, 44, *45*
  Spinach-Bacon Salad,
    60, 61
  Wilted Lettuce with Bacon,
    104
Bagel Thins, 14, *15*
Baked Chicken Thighs, 124,
    125
Baked Coffee Custard, 198
Baked Flounder with Tomato,
    176, 177

Balsamic Halibut, 178
Balsamic Vinaigrette, *91*, 93
Basil Pesto, 92
Beef. *See also* Lamb
  Beef Filet with Mushrooms,
    144
  Beef Pot Roast, *152*, 153
  Braised Short Ribs, *162*,
    163
  Cabbage and Ground Beef
    Soup, 38, *39*
  Cheeseburger Casserole,
    157
  Ginger Beef and
    Asparagus, 148, *149*
  Ground Beef and Cabbage,
    150
  No-Bean Chili, 35
  No-Noodle Lasagna, 154,
    155
  Pepper Steak, 151
  Rib-Eye Steaks in Red Wine
    Sauce, 142, *143*
  Steak Pinwheels, *158*, 159
  Stuffed Peppers, 156
  Zucchini Meatloaf, 145
Beverages, 209–218
  Almond Milk, 210
  Ginger-Turmeric Tea, *214*,
    218
  Golden Milk, 215
  Green Tea Smoothie, 211,
    213

Hot Cocoa, *214*, 215
Keto Coffee or Tea, 210
Raspberry Smoothie, 211,
    212–213
Strawberry Lemonade,
    216, *217*
Strawberry Milkshake, 216
Blue Cheese Dressing, 94
Bone Broth, Slow-Cooked
    Roasted, 26
Braised Short Ribs, *162*, 163
"Breaded" Flounder, 182,
    183
Breakfast, 1–23
  Almond Flour Pancakes,
    2, 3
  Bacon-Egg Cups, 10
  Bagel Thins, 14, *15*
  Breakfast Burrito, 20
  Breakfast Pizza, *22, 23*
  Broccoli-Cheddar Egg
    Muffins, 21
  Cauliflower "Mock"
    Porridge, 5
  Coconut–Almond Butter
    Bars, *12*, 13
  Coconut Flour Waffles,
    16, 17
  Egg Casserole with
    Sausage and Spinach,
    18, *19*
  Granola Cereal, 8, *9*
  Minute Muffin, 11

Breakfast (*continued*)
Scrambled Eggs with
Crabmeat, 4
Spinach-Tomato-Avocado
Omelet, *6, 7*
Broccoli
Broccoli and Cheese
Stuffed Chicken, *122, 123*
Broccoli-Cheddar Egg
Muffins, 21
Broccoli-Cheese Soup, 27
Broccoli Salad, 53, *54*
Chicken-Broccoli
Casserole, 121
Roasted Broccoli, 110, *112*
Brussels, Roasted, with
Bacon Soup, 44, *45*
Butter Fish, 180

C
Cabbage
Cabbage and Ground Beef
Soup, 38, *39*
Cabbage Salad, 65
Fried Cabbage with Bacon,
102, *103*
Ground Beef and Cabbage,
150
Sautéed Red Cabbage, 114
Casseroles
Cheeseburger Casserole,
157
Chicken-Broccoli
Casserole, 121
Egg Casserole with
Sausage and Spinach,
18, *19*
Tuna Casserole, 179
Cauliflower Mash, 105
Cauliflower "Mock" Porridge, 5
Celery, Sautéed, 107
Cheese, Almond, 72, *75*
Cheese (dairy)
Blue Cheese Dressing, 94
Broccoli and Cheese
Stuffed Chicken, *122, 123*

Broccoli-Cheese Soup, 27
Cheese Ball, 78
Cheeseburger Casserole,
157
Cheese Sauce, *91, 92*
Crustless Baked
Cheesecake, 186, *187*
Mexican Cheese Dip, 73
Raspberry-Cheese Muffins,
191
Chicken and turkey
Baked Chicken Thighs,
124, *125*
Broccoli and Cheese
Stuffed Chicken, *122,* 123
Chicken-Broccoli
Casserole, 121
Chicken Chili, *46,* 47
Chicken with Spinach and
Tomato, 137
Chicken Zoodle Soup, *30,*
31
Curried Chicken, *126,* 127
Filipino Chicken Adobo,
130, *131*
Garlic-Lemon Chicken, 120
Marinated Turkey
Tenderloins, 128
Pesto Chicken Salad, *66, 67*
Roasted Chicken, 118, *119*
Chili, Chicken, *46,* 47
Chili, No-Bean, 35
Chocolate
Chocolate Fudge Balls,
194, 195
Chocolate Mousse, 202,
203
Chocolate Sauce, 87
Hot Cocoa, *214,* 215
Clam Sauce, Creamy, Over
Zoodles, 181
Coconut
Coconut–Almond Butter
Bars, *12,* 13
Coconut Flour Waffles,
16, 17

Coconut Macaroons, 192,
193
Coconut Milk Pudding, 199
Coffee, Keto, 210
Coffee Custard, Baked, 198
Collard Greens, Ham and,
132, 133
Crabmeat, Scrambled Eggs
with, 4
Crab Quiche, *168,* 169
Cream, Fluffy Strawberry,
188, 189
Creamed Spinach, 114
Cream of Mushroom Soup,
40
Creamy Avocado Soup, *36, 37*
Creamy Clam Sauce Over
Zoodles, 181
Creamy Dill-Cucumber
Salad, 52
Crustless Baked Cheesecake,
186, *187*
Cucumbers
Creamy Dill-Cucumber
Salad, 52
Salmon-Cucumber Salad,
64
Stuffed Cucumber Slices,
77
Curried Chicken, *126,* 127
Custard, Baked Coffee, 198.
See also Pudding

D
Desserts, 185–207
Almond Butter Cookies,
200, 201
Almond Butter Cups, 206,
207
Almond Flour Cake, *204,*
205
Baked Coffee Custard, 198
Chocolate Fudge Balls,
194, 195
Chocolate Mousse, 202,
203

Coconut Macaroons, 192,
193
Coconut Milk Pudding, 199
Crustless Baked
Cheesecake, 186, *187*
Fluffy Strawberry Cream,
188, 189
No-Churn Vanilla Ice
Cream, 196, *197*
Quick Ricotta Pudding,
195
Raspberry-Cheese Muffins,
191
Vanilla Custard Pudding,
190
Dip, Mexican Cheese, 73
Dip, Sour Cream and Onion,
82, 83
Dressings and sauces,
85–95
Avocado Dressing, 86, *91*
Avocado Mayonnaise, 89
Balsamic Vinaigrette,
91, 93
Basil Pesto, 92
Blue Cheese Dressing, 94
Cheese Sauce, *91, 92*
Chocolate Sauce, 87
Italian Dressing, 86, *90*
Low-Carb Ketchup, 95
Maple Syrup, 88
Strawberry Sauce, 87, *90*

E
Egg Roll in a Bowl, 134, *135*
Eggs
Avocado Deviled Eggs,
74, 79
Bacon-Egg Cups, 10
Breakfast Pizza, *22, 23*
Broccoli-Cheddar Egg
Muffins, 21
Crab Quiche, *168,* 169
Egg Casserole with
Sausage and Spinach,
18, *19*

Egg Drop Soup, 32, *33*
Scrambled Eggs with
 Crabmeat, 4

F

Filipino Chicken Adobo, 130,
 131
Fish, Butter, 180
Fish Florentine, 166
Flounder, Baked, with
 Tomato, *176*, 177
Flounder, "Breaded," 182, *183*
Fluffy Strawberry Cream,
 188, 189
Fried Cabbage with Bacon,
 102, *103*
Fried Spinach with
 Mushrooms, 98, *99*
Fries, Turnip, 106

G

Garlicky Steamed Mussels,
 174, *175*
Garlic Lamb Chops, 160, *161*
Garlic-Lemon Chicken, 120
Ginger Beef and Asparagus,
 148, *149*
Ginger-Turmeric Tea, *214*, 218
Golden Milk, 215
Granola Cereal, 8, *9*
Green Bean–Tomato Salad,
 62, *63*
Green Tea Smoothie, 211, *213*
Ground Beef and Cabbage,
 150

H

Halibut, Balsamic, 178
Ham and Collard Greens,
 132, 133
Hot Cocoa, *214*, 215

I

Ice Cream, No-Churn Vanilla,
 196, *197*
Italian Dressing, 86, *90*

K

Kale, Baby, Salad, 58
Kale Soup, Sausage-, 28, *29*
Keto Coffee or Tea, 210

L

Lamb
 Garlic Lamb Chops, 160,
  161
 Lamb Patties, *146*, 147
Lasagna, No-Noodle, 154, *155*
Low-Carb Ketchup, 95

M

Main dishes. *See* Beef;
 Chicken and turkey;
 Lamb; Pork; Seafood
Maple Syrup, 88
Marinated Turkey
 Tenderloins, 128
Mexican Cheese Dip, 73
Minute Muffin, 11
"Mock" Porridge, Cauliflower, 5
Muffins
 Broccoli-Cheddar Egg
  Muffins, 21
 Minute Muffin, 11
 Raspberry-Cheese Muffins,
  191
Mushrooms
 Beef Filet with Mushrooms,
  144
 Cream of Mushroom
  Soup, 40
 Fried Spinach with
  Mushrooms, 98, *99*
 Mushrooms Provençale,
  107
Mussels, Garlicky Steamed,
 174, *175*

N

No-Bean Chili, 35
No-Churn Vanilla Ice Cream,
 196, *197*
No-Noodle Lasagna, 154, *155*

Nuts. *See also* Almonds
 Nutty Crackers, *75*, 76
 Walnut Zucchini, *112–113*,
  115

O

Oyster Stew, 34

P

Peppers
 Pepper Steak, 151
 Stir-Fried Squash and
  Pepper, *100*, 101
 Stuffed Peppers, 156
Pesto Chicken Salad, *66*, 67
Pizza, Breakfast, *22*, 23
Pork
 Egg Casserole with
  Sausage and Spinach,
  18, *19*
 Egg Roll in a Bowl, 134, *135*
 Pork Fried Rice, *108*, 109
 Pork Loin Roast, 136
 Quick "Breaded" Pork, *138*,
  139
 Sausage-Kale Soup, 28, *29*
 Smothered Pork Chops, 129
Poultry. *See* Chicken and
 turkey
Pudding
 Coconut Milk Pudding, 199
 Quick Ricotta Pudding, 195
 Vanilla Custard Pudding,
  190
Pumpkin Soup, 41

Q

Quiche, Crab, *168*, 169
Quick "Breaded" Pork, *138*,
 139
Quick Ricotta Pudding, 195

R

Radish Salad, *55*, 56
Raspberry-Cheese Muffins,
 191

Raspberry Smoothie, 211,
 212–213
Rib-Eye Steaks in Red Wine
 Sauce, 142, *143*
Roasted Broccoli, 110, *112*
Roasted Brussels with Bacon
 Soup, 44, *45*
Roasted Chicken, 118, *119*

S

Salads, 49–67
 Baby Kale Salad, 58
 Baby Vegetable Mixed
  Salad, 50, *51*
 Broccoli Salad, 53, *54*
 Cabbage Salad, 65
 Creamy Dill-Cucumber
  Salad, 52
 Green Bean–Tomato Salad,
  62, *63*
 Pesto Chicken Salad, *66*,
  67
 Radish Salad, *55*, 56
 Salmon-Cucumber Salad,
  64
 Sour Cream–Lettuce
  Salad, 57
 Spinach-Bacon Salad,
  60, 61
 Summer Squash Salad, 53,
  54–55
 Wedge Salad, 58
Salmon-Cucumber Salad, 64
Salmon with Creamy Dill
 Sauce, 166, *167*
Sauces. *See* Dressings and
 sauces
Sausage-Kale Soup, 28, *29*
Sautéed Celery, 107
Sautéed Red Cabbage, 114
Scrambled Eggs with
 Crabmeat, 4
Seafood, 165–183
 Baked Flounder with
  Tomato, *176*, 177
 Balsamic Halibut, 178

Seafood (*continued*)
"Breaded" Flounder, 182
Butter Fish, 180
Crab Quiche, *168*, 169
Creamy Clam Sauce Over Zoodles, 181
Fish Florentine, 166
Garlicky Steamed Mussels, 174, *175*
Salmon-Cucumber Salad, 64
Shrimp Scampi, 170, *171*
Stir-Fried Scallops, *172*, 173
Tuna Casserole, 179
Seasoned Tortilla Chips, 80, *81*
Side dishes, 97–115
Almond Asparagus, 111, *113*
Cauliflower Mash, 105
Creamed Spinach, 114
Fried Cabbage with Bacon, 102, *103*
Fried Spinach with Mushrooms, 98, *99*
Mushrooms Provençale, 107
Pork Fried Rice, *108*, 109
Roasted Broccoli, 110, *112*
Sautéed Celery, 107
Sautéed Red Cabbage, 114
Stir-Fried Squash and Pepper, *100*, 101
Turnip Fries, 106
Walnut Zucchini, *112–113*, 115
Wilted Lettuce with Bacon, 104

Slow-Cooked Roasted Bone Broth, 26
Smoothie, Green Tea, 211, *213*
Smoothie, Raspberry, 211, *212–213*
Smothered Pork Chops, 129
Soups and stews, 25–47
Broccoli-Cheese Soup, 27
Cabbage and Ground Beef Soup, 38, *39*
Chicken Chili, *46*, 47
Chicken Zoodle Soup, *30*, 31
Cream of Mushroom Soup, 40
Creamy Avocado Soup, *36*, 37
Egg Drop Soup, 32, *33*
No-Bean Chili, 35
Oyster Stew, 34
Pumpkin Soup, 41
Roasted Brussels with Bacon Soup, 44, *45*
Sausage-Kale Soup, 28, *29*
Slow-Cooked Roasted Bone Broth, 26
Yellow Squash Soup, *42*, 43
Sour Cream and Onion Dip, 82, 83
Sour Cream–Lettuce Salad, 57
Spinach
Chicken with Spinach and Tomato, 137
Creamed Spinach, 114

Egg Casserole with Sausage and Spinach, 18, *19*
Fish Florentine, 166
Fried Spinach with Mushrooms, 98, *99*
Spinach-Bacon Salad, *60*, 61
Spinach-Tomato-Avocado Omelet, *6*, 7
Squash
Chicken Zoodle Soup, *30*, 31
Pumpkin Soup, 41
Stir-Fried Squash and Pepper, *100*, 101
Summer Squash Salad, 53, *54–55*
Walnut Zucchini, *112–113*, 115
Yellow Squash Soup, *42*, 43
Zucchini Meatloaf, 145
Steak Pinwheels, *158*, 159
Stir-Fried Scallops, *172*, 173
Strawberries
Fluffy Strawberry Cream, *188*, 189
Strawberry Lemonade, 216, *217*
Strawberry Milkshake, 216
Strawberry Sauce, 87, *90*
Stuffed Cucumber Slices, 77
Stuffed Peppers, 156
Summer Squash Salad, 53, *54–55*

T
Tea
Ginger-Turmeric Tea, *214*, 218
Green Tea Smoothie, 211, *213*
Keto Tea, 210
Tortilla Chips, Seasoned, 80, *81*
Tuna Casserole, 179
Turkey Tenderloins, Marinated, 128
Turmeric
Ginger-Turmeric Tea, *214*, 218
Golden Milk, 215
Turnip Fries, 106

V
Vanilla Custard Pudding, 190
Vanilla Ice Cream, No-Churn, 196, *197*
Vegetable, Baby, Mixed Salad, 50, *51*
Vinaigrette, Balsamic, *91*, 93

W
Walnut Zucchini, *112–113*, 115
Wedge Salad, 58
Wilted Lettuce with Bacon, 104

Y
Yellow Squash Soup, *42*, 43

Z
Zucchini, Walnut, *112–113*, 115
Zucchini Meatloaf, 145